perimenopowei

# perimenopower

*Your Essential Guide to the Change
Before the Change*

## KATARINA WILK

Translated by Karin Shearman

First published in Sweden in 2018 by Ehrlin Publishing

First published in Great Britain in 2020 by Orion Spring
an imprint of The Orion Publishing Group Ltd
Carmelite House, 50 Victoria Embankment
London EC4Y 0DZ

An Hachette UK Company

1 3 5 7 9 10 8 6 4 2

A CIP catalogue record for this book is
available from the British Library.

ISBN (Trade Paperback) 978 1 4091 9854 3
ISBN (eBook) 978 1 4091 9855 0

Every effort has been made to ensure that the information in the book is accurate.
The information in this book may not be applicable in each individual case so it
is advised that professional medical advice is obtained for specific health matters
and before changing any medication or dosage. Neither the publisher nor author
accepts any legal responsibility for any personal injury or other damage or
loss arising from the use of the information in this book. In addition if you are
concerned about your diet or exercise regime and wish to change them, you should
consult a health practitioner first.

Printed and bound in Great Britain by
Clays Ltd, Elcograf S.p.A

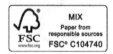

MIX
Paper from
responsible sources
FSC
www.fsc.org
FSC® C104740

www.orionbooks.co.uk

You just do it.
You just force yourself to get up.
You force yourself to put one foot in front of the other
and, God damn it,
you refuse to let it get to you.
You fight. You cry. You curse.
Then you go about the business of living.
That's how I've done it.
There is no other way.

*Elizabeth Taylor*

# Contents

# Introduction

A few years ago, strange things started happening to my body. I couldn't sleep and was experiencing panic attacks and sudden bouts of sweating. There were so many odd sensations happening all at once, and it made me sad and confused. Perhaps this is the way you feel right now? Worried and low? As if all you want is to get rid of this feeling, although you can barely explain what it is?

During a girls' dinner party, when I reluctantly admitted how I felt, everyone started laughing with recognition. In the end, we all laughed so hard that we cried. *Everyone* had similar symptoms, but none of us realised then that it might be because we were getting close to the time when our periods would stop. We still had regular cycles and we were only in our forties. We had heard that you could experience similar physical symptoms during the menopause, but surely that was something that happened when you were getting close to fifty? None of us had even heard of the perimenopause.

Being a curious person by nature, I decided to find out more, and realised that what we were going through was the perimenopause – the wild hormonal ride that leads up to the menopause, when your periods stop for good. When I saw how little collective knowledge there was about the subject and how many conflicting theories and pieces of advice were floating around, I decided to write this book. My whole working life has been spent as a writer and editor with a focus on health, wellness and medicine. I have always had a great interest in the amazing power of the female body: just the fact that a woman can carry and give birth to babies is incredible. Your body is a miracle and you need to look after it carefully, especially during sensitive transitions such as puberty, pregnancy and the perimenopause – times when your female sex hormones go crazy.

This book cannot replace professional health care by qualified doctors, and it is not intended to. If you feel really unwell you need to get professional help. I won't be saying that oestrogen is better than natural medicines or that cardio training is better than strength training. Instead, I will present different alternatives and solutions, and give you the option of making an informed decision for your own body and your own needs. I am offering you a chance to take charge of your life and I hope you will realise that you don't have to live with these symptoms if you don't want to.

You are not a hostage to your hormones – you have the power to make changes that will help you to feel better.

The one thing I can promise is that I have tried every possible treatment for the perimenopause, and today I am in better physical and mental shape than ever. But it has been a long and winding road, and it is this journey that I want to share with you. There is a huge lack of knowledge about the perimenopause, but I hope that this book will help to break the silence.

Between you and me, most of my friends are 'patients' of mine. I am known in my group of girls as the one who pretends to be a doctor. At the first sign of a symptom, I try to help them as best I can with the knowledge I have. Even if it's just to support them there and then. I want to help you too. I want you to feel more secure after reading this book. I hope you will understand more about what is going on inside your body and how to turn the negatives into positives. This period in your life isn't an illness, it's simply a phase – a phase that affects most women in the world and will not last for ever.

I want to make you feel that you are not alone with your symptoms, and also inform you about what happens in the female body. For example, did you know that the hormonal transitions that occur before your last period can go on for as long as ten to fifteen years before your periods finally stop? Most of the symptoms you have are not unusual or alarming; they are simply the result of your hormones being completely off track.

The first part of this book is based upon my own experiences, which you may recognise in yourself. To make it easier for you, I will guide you through the necessary medical terms and describe what is going on inside your body. The second part of the book is about what you can do in order to feel your best. My hope is that you will use this book as a guide on your journey to find your superpower when your hormones start to fluctuate.

*Perimenopower* is for those of you who are thirty-five and older and interested in understanding why you are sleepless, sweaty and feeling down. It's for anyone who wants to get the best tips for waking up well rested, fresh and happy. I want to help you find yourself again. You could say that the book is the result of my own extremely difficult hormonal storms in combination with a somewhat obsessive interest in medicine. All medical facts have been checked by Evelina Sande Idenfeldt, who is a senior doctor in gynaecology and obstetrics.

'Perimenopower' is a word that I invented to convey what it is possible for all of us who are experiencing this transition to achieve. You do not have to be a victim of your hormonal changes. You can be the heroine of this transition instead. To be a woman is, in itself, a superpower, and perimenopower is exactly what you need to get through this difficult phase. This power is already inside you, but with all of these strange symptoms you may feel that it has vanished out of sight. This book is here to remind you that are incredibly strong, even if you feel that your strength has disappeared. Try to remember all those hard times in your life when all you wanted to do was to curl up in a little ball and shut out the world. You may have done just that for a while, but you always managed to get up again and keep going. Use that strength now. Your perimenopower is there, I promise. And I will help you find it.

*Katarina Wilk*

**Perimenopause:** the time before your final period when hormonal changes are experienced. It can start as early as thirty-five, but for most women it begins between the ages of forty and forty-five.

# PART ONE

# What Is the Perimenopause?

# 1

# My Story

'I was getting so desperate from lack of
sleep that I felt almost suicidal.'

**KATARINA, FORTY-THREE**

**Insomnia:** the medical term for sleeplessness. It means that you are unable to sleep, you sleep badly or wake early. It can be temporary or more sustained.

My first symptoms began soon after I turned forty. Why did I feel so low? Why was I unable to sleep? Why did I wake at night with palpitations and sheets drenched in sweat? I didn't know where to turn, or even if my symptoms were anything to be taken seriously. I could hardly explain the sensations even to myself, and I didn't know if they were related or separate or if maybe I was just going crazy. All I knew was that I needed to find answers.

## I'm not depressed – I just want to sleep

I remember it vividly. It was just before Christmas and I simply could not get to sleep. It wasn't that I had difficulties going to sleep or that I woke up several times in the night. I didn't sleep a wink, not even one second, throughout the night. Have you ever experienced this? If you have then you know that the only thing you think about when you can't sleep is how much you want to sleep. This in turn builds up panic and frustration, which makes falling asleep less likely than ever.

At first, I explained away the sleeplessness as stress. You know how it is around Christmas. There's food to be cooked, presents to be bought and trips to grandparents and in-laws to be planned. We all have a thousand things on our minds and it's hard to switch off. But in the end the sleeplessness got so bad that I went to my doctor, who asked if I was finding things difficult at the moment. Was I feeling low? I had to stop myself from shoving the stethoscope down her throat. Of course I felt low, most people who get no sleep feel low! It was the wrong question, and she offered me no solution. I was starting to panic. I felt so bad and I was getting no help. And I simply couldn't get to sleep.

A day or two later, I returned to the medical centre and started to cry out of sheer hopelessness. The doctor realised that I had to be helped or something terrible would happen, so she prescribed some strong sleeping tablets. 'It's either depression or exhaustion,' she said, and, despite feeling neither depressed nor exhausted, I nodded while sobbing. I had no other alternative.

I took one of the strong sleeping pills that same evening. But it was the first, and definitely the last, time I went down that route. I suffered terrible hallucinations, and what should have been beauty sleep ended with me hardly daring to go to sleep again. The nightmares I had that night were worse than all the horror films I'd ever seen put together. So much blood, so many babies without heads. When I woke, I was completely wiped out and filled with such anxiety that I thought I may need admitting to a psychiatric unit.

So, although I'd been asleep, it was a sleep I could have done without. On my next visit to the medical centre I told the doctor about my night filled with nightmares.

'I think you should start a course of antidepressants, you show all the signs of being depressed,' said the doctor. I have since learned that this is a very common diagnosis given to women who are experiencing perimenopausal symptoms.

'I don't want to take antidepressants,' I begged. 'I'm not depressed, I just want to sleep. It must be something else.'

'It's probably just temporary, continue with the sleeping tablets and you'll be fine. These things just happen some-times,' the doctor said.

I was terribly sad when I left her office. My questions about why I felt the way I did had not been answered; instead it was as though the doctor had tried to persuade me that I was depressed even though I didn't feel like that at all. I was more confused when I left than when I had arrived.

## Seeing connections and looking for solutions

Once Christmas was over, we went to Spain. I was feeling panicked, since I still didn't know why my body refused to sleep. The panic grew every day as I got more and more tired. I simply could not get to sleep. But I had lived in

France during my youth and I knew that you could get strong medicines over the counter in southern Europe – and I was not disappointed.

The local pharmacist in the Andalusian mountain village recommended a supplement of melatonin, a natural sleep hormone that is produced by the body but which decreases with age. Melatonin is sold in Europe and the US but not in Sweden. I had taken it a few years earlier for sleeping problems caused by jetlag and it had worked then.

I took some over-the-counter melatonin and finally I could begin to sleep a little again. But I still wondered what was going on: my brain was working overtime. My natural curiosity told me it was important to understand what caused the sleeplessness – it felt like a symptom of something, and not the main problem for me.

I had also started to suffer from low blood sugar, and had to eat regularly in order not to feel weak and shaky. I had never experienced it so vividly before. Have you had problems with blood sugar? If you have, you will know how faint you can suddenly feel. As if you want to devour an entire bar of chocolate just to get some energy back.

Then I suddenly realised that during the past autumn I had also suffered panic attacks and at times felt pressure across my chest, as if my body was constantly tense and I couldn't relax. I had never felt this before; it was completely new to me. Where did this unease come from?

Sometimes I awoke from paranoid nightmares completely sweat-soaked, with a racing pulse. I felt seriously ill and worried. Has this happened to you too?

I refused to accept the doctor's theories of exhaustion and depression and instead I wanted to find solutions to my problems aside from sleeping pills and antidepressants. I was determined to find answers myself, or at least find out what options were available to help me. I felt I was on a mission, not just for myself but for everyone else in this situation: if I could find what worked for me, perhaps I could then help others too.

I want to clarify once again that the perimenopause isn't an illness but a phase that most women go through. Some of us suffer more, others less, and sometimes it's hard to say which came first, the chicken or the egg. Do you get anxious from not sleeping, or do you not sleep because you are anxious? In the end, it doesn't really matter. You need to take what you are experiencing seriously, and not just accept living with symptoms that can be cured relatively easily.

Eventually I found straightforward solutions that reduced all my symptoms, including sweating, feeling low and sleeplessness. It was almost a shock to discover how simply these issues could be dealt with, once I knew what was happening to me. I hope the following pages will help you find your own way back to feeling like yourself again.

**Hot flush/flash:** a sudden and intense sensation of heat experienced by some women during the perimenopause and menopause. May be accompanied by perspiration and a rapid heartbeat. Hot flushes can last between two and thirty minutes, and can occur multiple times during the day and night. Hot flushes at night are known as night sweats.

# 2

# You Are Not Alone

'When I had my first hot flush at night and googled night sweats, I was terrified. Then I told my boss and she just laughed in recognition.'

**LINN, FORTY-FOUR**

I have always been fascinated by the human body. So many different systems have to work in sync for our bodies to function optimally, and most of the time they actually do. We just expect our bodies to come along for the ride while we get on with our important business of work, family and other responsibilities. If you're used to generally feeling well, it can be very hard to realise that your body no longer works perfectly. It's not coming along for the ride any more; instead it's slowing down to a halt. That was how I felt, anyhow.

I am not a hypochondriac and am rarely ill, so when my body began to go on strike and strange symptoms, both physical and mental, appeared from nowhere it felt very odd. What is going on? Why do I feel so peculiar? No one had warned me about this.

## We are all in the same boat

I started to research my symptoms online, in books and in medical research papers. I watched every TV interview I could find and ploughed through podcasts in search of the slightest recognition. I began to realise that I was encountering something that simply wasn't spoken about. Not with your friends, your husband or even your doctor. You are not supposed to talk about sweaty nights, insomnia or panic attacks.

If you ask your mother about the perimenopause, she may say that she never had any problems at all, or that she doesn't remember. It is hard to find anyone of the older generation willing to discuss it openly. My theory is that the subject is either taboo, in that it's too personal to talk about, or that many women never connect their symptoms with hormonal changes if those symptoms appear when they are young as thirty-five to forty years of age.

With a little luck, you have a mother who remembers how it was for her and supports you through it. Many hormonal issues can be hereditary. If your mother had problems, you may have similar ones. If she only had difficulty in sleeping and nothing else, it's plausible that you too will only suffer from sleep issues.

When my mother was still alive I asked her about how she felt during the menopause. She couldn't remember having any discomforts at all. Perhaps she belonged to the group of mothers who don't want to talk about these things and, naturally, this must be respected. But do ask your mother if you get the chance. It can give you a hint of what is to come, and the chances are that she has valuable tips and hints about what worked for her. Bear in mind, though, that she belongs to a different generation, which means that she may have opinions that you don't agree with. Things will have changed culturally since she went through her own transition, and medical knowledge and advice will have advanced over the years too.

But please do remember that there is nothing wrong with you. Don't panic that you have been hit by a dangerous disease or that you're experiencing something that's not normal. When you know what you're going through, you'll see that many others have shared your symptoms and dealt with them.

Now that I have started to talk openly about my problems and written a book about the perimenopause, most of my friends have recognised that they are having symptoms themselves. They range from my little sister, who has just turned forty-two, telling me that she feels a bit low sometimes for no apparent reason, to my colleague who is thirty-seven and cannot sleep. My initial perception was that talking about the subject with girlfriends was like walking on thin ice, but now that we're open about how we're feeling our dinners are more fun than ever; often my stomach aches from too much laughter. Try bringing up the subject with your friends; the chances are that you will laugh and cry at the same time at everyone's stories. The community that emerges when women are open and honest can support and uplift you through the perimenopause if you just dare to start talking about it.

I also feel closer to the women at work since we started talking about the strange things we had been experiencing. A good friend of mine told me how she had been dating a new man who asked her in the middle of the night whether she wanted some medicine to relieve her fever. What do you think her date would have thought if she'd told the truth? 'I didn't have a fever last night, I am just entering the menopause.'

## It's hard to see the whole picture

When I went to the doctor that first time about my perimenopausal symptoms, I felt that no one was listening to me or taking me seriously. They thought they knew what was going on in my body, but I realised they were talking nonsense. I don't know if it comes down to a lack of knowledge on the part of medical professionals or if they don't believe the symptoms even exist. But, as any woman can tell you, they very much do.

Of course, it can sometimes be difficult to see that these symptoms are connected when, individually, they can have many different reasons, and in small doses they might not even appear abnormal or strange. But I wish that the connection between them and hormonal changes could be made before doctors prescribe sleeping pills and antidepressants. If you are over thirty-five, your doctor should ask you about your menstrual cycle instead of assuming that you are suffering from exhaustion. He or she should ask about your sleeping patterns and if you have anxiety or hot flushes at night. And, when they have managed to understand what is going on, the first step should be to refer you to a gynaecologist, who is a specialist in the female, hormone-filled body.

Some gynaecologists want to measure your hormone levels, while others interpret your hormonal changes by looking at your symptoms. Once I realised my problems may be hormonal and visited my gynaecologist, it was like a weight being lifted off my shoulders. She looked at me and smiled and said that she would sort me out. This was the first time I heard that my symptoms had something to do with the menopause. No one had told me before that hormones can change for a long time before your periods stop. One of the positives of visiting my gynaecologist was that I had already been seeing her for several years. She had followed me from pregnancy to perimenopause, and knew what was normal for me and what was not. It was a great relief to talk to someone with the experience and ability to put into words these things that I had never encountered before.

She asked me to keep a diary of my symptoms, and I strongly suggest that you do this too if you are feeling overwhelmed by all the changes you are going through. I began taking notes every time I experienced something that might be related to hormonal imbalance. By looking at my records over the days and weeks, my gynaecologist could determine that the symptoms were hormonal and linked to my menstrual cycle and nothing else. I have an awful lot to thank this woman for.

Access to a trusted gynaecologist who knows your history is something that I wish all women had. It really helps. Ask your gynaecologist to explain the symptoms and their causes to you in a simple-to-understand way. Perhaps you lack the energy to investigate this yourself, or simply don't want to absorb everything in as much detail as I do, with my obsessive interest in anything to do with the body. But try to understand the basics. It will make things a lot easier for you, and help you to explain your symptoms to your doctor or other medical professionals. I will give you a head start on the basic terminology in the next chapter.

**Anxiety:** an emotion characterised by unpleasant sensations of distress or fear, often accompanied by nervous behaviour. May include feelings of dread over imminent events.

# 3

# Understanding the Terminology

'What do you mean, the menopause? I had just turned thirty-eight, had no children and was suddenly having daily panic attacks. I was completely convinced that I was very ill.'

**ANNA, THIRTY-EIGHT**

What enters your mind when you hear the term 'meno-pause'? Apart from finding it a negatively charged term, and one that most people would rather not discuss, to many it is also surrounded by confusion. If you ask your female friends what it means, most will probably say it is when your periods end at around the age of fifty. If you ask them how long the run-up to the menopause lasts, most will have no clue. Most people seem to reckon that they might experience a few symptoms around the age of fifty, and the majority believe that the menopause is the begin-ning of the end of your life as a fertile, vibrant woman. Perhaps many of us would rather not think, in our prime years, that the symptoms we are experiencing are related to hormones and ageing. That might mean we are starting to get old.

We fear getting old – that can't be denied. Personally, I would like to have stayed thirty-five for the rest of my life. But getting older is inevitable, and I think it's time that we start to see that there is a power and a wisdom in ageing. I believe if we don't embrace this change, it can only be our own fault if the term 'menopause' is so negative. Age doesn't have to be something unattractive.

I mean, have you seen Elon Musk's mother? Maye Musk still works as a supermodel in her seventies. Google her. She is one of the most beautiful women I've ever seen, and she is beautiful because of her age and not in spite of it.

Not many people in their mid-thirties imagine that the symptoms they are experiencing might be to do with hormones. It is more common to blame work stress, or relationship issues, or the demands of a family life. In the same way, it is often difficult for doctors to join up the dots. Instead, we waste time looking for other diagnoses because we don't have sufficient knowledge about hormonal problems or how much of a woman's life is affected by them.

If you look up the word 'menopause' online, you might get confused. The International Menopause Society (IMS) stated as long ago as 1999 that there was a misuse of terminology related to this field among healthcare providers, media and the public which was bewildering. There is a great deal of misunderstanding – even among medical professionals – about the difference between the perimenopause and the menopause.

Some medical professionals use the term 'climacteric' for the time when a woman's periods stop completely, but this is a confusing definition and is not commonly used these days. The climacteric actually refers to the transition leading up to the menopause – the perimenopause.

I find it easiest to explain the distinction as follows:

## Perimenopause

From the Greek, where *peri* means around. In other words, the word *peri* + menopause means the time around the menopause. The perimenopause is not a single point in time, but a period of transition during which you will still be having menstrual cycles. As hormones fluctuate, your cycles may become less frequent and the length of your cycles may change. This is the transition that we are exploring in *Perimenopower*.

There is no universal age for when the hormones start changing, but normally the symptoms are experienced between the ages of forty and fifty. They can come as early as thirty-five. We are all different, but for most people they can go on for several years. The purpose of this book is to help you through the perimenopause, regardless of whether you enter it two or fifteen years before your periods stop.

Some people refer to the 'premenopause' to refer to this time in a woman's life, but this is not a helpful term and is not used by medical professionals. I prefer to stick to the definition of the perimenopause.

## Menopause

From the French *menèspausie*, where *menès* means monthly and *pausie* means to end.

When you have not had your period for twelve consecutive months you are said to have reached the menopause, the time when your periods have stopped completely. The perimenopause is over and you are on the other side, where you don't need to think about sanitary towels or contraceptives. It's the period-free side where you can no longer bear children.

Some people find it difficult when their periods stop, while others are elated. Some slip into existential depression and, of course, this is a passage in life that makes you think. Regardless of whether you have had children or not, the menopause is a sign that your reproductive life is over. You have no more chances to produce a biological offspring. I understand why this makes many people feel low, for after all, childbirth is among the greatest things that can happen in one's life; but at the same time, think about all the other things life can offer. So don't despair if you find it difficult to handle the changes you are facing. We will sort this out.

**Panic attack:** a sudden period of intense fear that may be accompanied by heart palpitations, sweating, shaking, shortness of breath and numbness. In some cases panic attacks cause chest pain that can be mistaken for a heart attack.

# 4

# What's Wrong with Our Bodies?

'I would do anything to feel like myself again.
It's intolerable to feel this way for so long.'

**LISA, FORTY-FIVE**

Despite the advances of medical science, the human body is in many ways still a big, beautiful mystery, and one of its greatest mysteries is the role of hormones. They affect our metabolism, reproductive ability, sexual maturity, libido and many other things.

The hormonal system is made up of endocrine glands. These glands produce hormones, which you can think of as chemical messengers that take their instructions to different parts of the body. They are transported via your blood like small armies with specific goals. These hormones have many special skills, and we certainly don't know all of them yet. Some are experts at reducing stress, others make sure your body grows and develops as it's programmed to. One thing's for sure: hormones are very determined and highly skilled at their job. Just like people who are experts in their field, hormones know exactly what they are supposed to do.

A well-known hormone that has gained superstar status in the world of health is insulin. Insulin wins first prize when it comes to lowering your blood-sugar level. After devouring a packet of sweets, insulin works hard to take care of that sugar for you.

However, if you have a uterus, the hormones that are your best friends – and sometimes your worst enemies, which we will return to later – are the female sex hormones, oestrogen and progesterone. They are sometimes known as ovarian hormones, since they have their headquarters in your ovaries. They are the ones that ensure you have your period every month and that your body can develop a baby should your egg be fertilised.

But, as with a best friend, there may be times when the two of you don't completely agree, and even though oestrogen and progesterone normally work *for* you, suddenly they may start causing trouble. You enter the perimenopause when your balance of oestrogen and progesterone begin to change and fluctuate. Your hormones start acting like unruly teenagers going bananas, leaving you completely unable to predict what they will do next.

The reason you feel unwell during this period is that the level of sex hormones changes. There is unease in the hormone camp. You could liken the fluctuating hormones to a dance. When you are feeling well it's largely thanks to your hormones. When you are feeling ill it's also often because of your hormones. Your sex hormones dance around in your body and their relationship with each other affects your entire being.

Do you remember the movie *Dirty Dancing*? It's not until the main characters are completely in sync with each other that they are able to accomplish the lift at the end. For you to be best able to help your body, it's good to understand that what's going on with your hormones affects your whole well-being. Which is exactly what happens with the characters in *Dirty Dancing*: when they are in harmony, the dance goes well. When your hormones work together in harmony, you feel well.

So, now I would like to give you a deeper insight into how sex hormones work. I do appreciate that you may find it hard to grasp all of this, but try to glean as much insight as you need in order to better understand your body.

## The basis of the menstrual cycle

In order to describe what happens to the hormones during the perimenopause, we first need to look at a normal menstrual cycle. And, without complicating matters more than is necessary, here follows a basic description of how the hormones work in a typical menstrual cycle.

A menstrual cycle lasts an average of twenty-eight days. For some the cycle is as short as twenty-five days and for others it can be longer. During a menstrual cycle, the levels of oestrogen and progesterone vary. Some days the difference is greater, and this is what makes you notice an imbalance in your body which can manifest itself physically or mentally.

The menstrual cycle is counted from the first day of your period to the first day of your next period. At the beginning and the end of the cycle, levels of both oestrogen and progesterone are low. One week after your period starts, oestrogen levels begin to rise, while progesterone levels remain at the same level a while longer. Approximately two weeks after your period, oestrogen levels peak while progesterone levels are slowly gathering speed. After this, you are ovulating. This is the time at which your body is its most fertile and you are ready to conceive. You could say that the ovulation in the middle of your menstrual cycle is the climax of that cycle. The progesterone reaches its top level and the oestrogen starts to dip.

During the last week before your period, the levels of both oestrogen and progesterone decrease. Finally, you will have your period and your menstrual cycle will begin all over again. In other words, you regularly experience substantial changes in hormone levels while you still bleed regularly. But these changes are normal and, importantly, they are the same every menstrual cycle.

When you enter the perimenopause, it no longer works that way. Instead your hormones begin to act more like headless chickens, running around with no sense of direction. They do not follow each other predictably like they used to, when the 'hormone dance' worked as normal. All of a sudden, one is pulling away from the other uncontrollably while the other is fighting back and your body is starting to become very unsettled. Just as in *Dirty Dancing*, when they are not in sync the dance doesn't work.

## Progesterone levels drop

The first hormone to decrease during the perimenopause is progesterone. Many of the symptoms that arise are caused by lower progesterone levels. Or, to be more accurate, the symptoms result from a reduced progesterone level in combination with a stable oestrogen level. We are simply getting too little progesterone in relation to how much oestrogen we have left. The normal changes that we have during our menstrual cycle are completely disrupted.

Hormone changes are natural, but when they start changing in a way that's unnatural in relation to each other, then hormone chaos ensues. During the perimenopause, the sex hormones refuse to work together in the way they have always done before. It may feel as if they are acting unpredictably and we must help them to find each other again. Because if your hormones find peace, so will you.

## Severe PMS that never ends

Perhaps you have suffered from PMS at some time in your life? PMS is an abbreviation for premenstrual syndrome and it usually occurs one to seven days before your period, as a result of an imbalance in your hormones. Some women are more susceptible to the hormonal imbalance and experience PMS more acutely than others.

The symptoms of PMS can be both physical and mental. Do you have tender breasts before your period? This is typical of PMS. Or do you feel really low, crying at the slightest thing? This is also common with PMS. Many people liken the perimenopause to intense and constant PMS. Perimenopause differs from PMS in that it feels as if it never ends. After all, PMS has a beginning and an end, and normally limits itself to a maximum of one week per month. The PMS-like problems can also be experienced more severely during the perimenopause.

You can also see similarities between the perimenopause and other times in life when your hormones are disrupted. For example, if you found it difficult going through puberty and pregnancy, you run a greater risk of being affected during the perimenopause as well. But if you danced your way through these hormonal transitions without major problems, there is less chance that you will have problems now.

My gynaecologist always tells me that it's no wonder I had problems during the perimenopause since I have also experienced severe PMS. Some people are simply more sensitive to hormonal changes than others. What do you think will happen in your case? Do you remember your puberty? If so, you might see similarities with what you are going through now, or even be able to predict what lies ahead.

## High sensitivity

I also believe that there are other causes that affect how sensitive you are to hormonal unease. Some women tend to be more sensitive to *everything* than others. Can you see a pattern among your group of friends? Is there anyone who is more sensitive and generally more affected by what's going on around them than others?

Have you heard about HSP? It stands for 'highly sensitive person' and means that you have a very sensitive personality and experience things at a higher, or subtler, level than other people. In other words, you have a more finely tuned system for picking up signals and sensory impressions that others might not notice. Imagine if, as an HSP, you sense your hormones more than other people?

I myself am a hormonally sensitive person and probably have a slight slant towards HSP. I have big feelings and take in everything that goes on around me. But during this period when I felt so unwell, I pulled myself together for the first time in a long while. I refused to accept that just because I am highly sensitive I would have a breakdown over a bunch of strange symptoms.

I thought about my children, how hard it can be to watch your happy mum not being so happy any longer. I thought about my puberty, when I felt really awful. For their sake and my own, I therefore tried to change my mindset about this transitional time of life. Of course, I still have times or days when I am not at my best, but overall I feel increasingly better with age and I believe much of it is about attitude. A psychologist friend of mine often says that she thinks I have developed a strong resistance, that nowadays I can remain upright even in stormy weather.

What I am trying to say is that, regardless of how sensitive you are to hormonal changes, I am convinced that you can improve your situation and work on your resistance, even if much of it is genetic. I believe I am a pretty good example of this, and maybe you will be too if you try following my advice. I hope that I'll be able to help you and that there is information in the following chapters that will make you feel better.

**Feeling emotional:** oestrogen acts as a mild antidepressant in the body and generally keeps us feeling content. When oestrogen levels drop during the perimenopause it is common for us to feel more emotional, weepy or sensitive.

# 5

# What Is Happening?

'I started a new job and was crushed by a total lack of self-confidence, despite years of experience. I almost resigned over it, before realising my anxiety was related to my hormones, rather than my abilities at work.'

**ANNA, FORTY-SIX**

By now, you know that the perimenopausal symptoms I am describing are due to the fact that the hormones are starting to change. These fluctuations happen to most women but affect us to different degrees. The amount of hormonal problems you experience can also depend upon where in the world you live. Factors like diet, lifestyle and climate may affect us more than we think, and the symptoms may not just be dependent on our physiology – that is, how our bodies work.

## Different symptoms in different parts of the world

PubMed is a database with over 30 million medical-related references to studies which are sometimes used as a basis for wider research. It's like an enormous digital library covering the world's medical studies.

In 2014, a major examination of the sixty-four most important studies in PubMed covering the symptoms apparent in perimenopause was conducted by a Polish team. The idea of this study was to investigate how perimenopausal symptoms differ in various parts of the world.

The results proved very interesting. In the United States, aching joints and muscles were most common. Australian women suffered more than others from vasomotor symptoms (those that are to do with the blood vessels' ability to expand and contract, e.g. hot flushes and sweating) and sexual dysfunction. In Africa there was no clear pattern; instead several different symptoms were prominent. In Europe, sleeping problems and depression weighed heaviest, and Asian women generally had milder symptoms than those in other parts of the world.

I find it fascinating that there are geographical and cultural differences in how the menopause is experienced around the world. Why do you think this is?

The Polish study did not reach any conclusion as to *why* the symptoms varied for different groups of women around the world, but it's probable that lifestyle has an influence. Diet and cultural habits relating to physical activity may have something to do with it. An average Westerner may exercise at the gym for a couple of hours per week, while elsewhere you may have to walk for an hour each day to fetch water.

I also believe that the way we see ourselves differs. In some countries age is associated with authority, while in the West we have a very deep-rooted youth culture where we do everything in our power not to grow old. 'Growing old' is still seen as something negative, and this perception affects women more than men as we are considered to be of less value once we are no longer fertile. This is particularly apparent in the beauty industry, which markets all sorts of potions and treatments aimed at making us look younger. In such a culture it's no wonder that nearing the menopause is seen as the beginning of the end for us women.

When women discuss the menopause, I often get the feeling that we come at it from the position of martyrs. Often we complain about this symptom and that, inviting people to feel sorry for us. What if we could turn things around and instead choose to see ageing as something liberating? What if we could view this as the start of a new chapter in life that we should feel grateful to experience? Think about this when you are feeling low – is it you or the society you live in that makes you feel bad?

As I mentioned earlier, sleep is one of the crucial things for well-being, but your self-image is equally important during this period. Society may have told you that you must stay young, but you can choose to embrace ageing. Do as the Maya Indians did: despite the various discomforting symptoms, women in their culture looked forward to the menopause. It meant a sense of freedom from child-rearing and a higher social status. In India, as early as the 1970s, this period in a woman's life was described as one which would give her new social possibilities, like laughing and joking with men in public.

Although it's rather sad that in these cultures women did not reach the same status as men until they stopped having periods every month, it's an example of how the perception of women is associated with the menopause. Whereas in the Western world we are told that we should be young and beautiful and that the menopause stops us from being so, in some countries it's a symbol of new-won freedom. I think we should be grateful for ageing; many people never get the chance to grow old. Just being alive is a gift. Don't ever forget that. Find your perimenopower and feel more free and beautiful than ever.

## What are we suffering from?

So what *is* on this smorgasbord of perimenopausal symptoms? Well, the list is long and varies from woman to woman. But there are some symptoms that appear more frequently than others. How about irregular periods, unusually heavy bleeding or spotting, sleeplessness, weight gain, hot flushes, palpitations, night sweats, mood swings, headaches, incontinence, dry mucus membranes, reduced sex drive, joint and muscle pain, tiredness, anxiety, depression and panic attacks. Doesn't it make you sweaty just reading about it? The first symptom is normally a change in your bleeding pattern: your periods become more frequent or infrequent than before.

With the help of this book I want to help you become well rested, fresh and alert. Then you will find the key to your superpower. First, I will go through some of the things that occur in your body when you are sleepless, sweaty and down in the dumps.

## Hot flushes – like having a bucket of warm juice poured over you

I will never forget the first time I had a hot flush. I was in a meeting and I felt as though I was about to have a panic attack. First, a wave of anxiety came over me; soon after that I had a feeling of warmth in my upper body and I began to have severe cold sweats. Have you ever woken up in the middle of the night with sweat pouring down your whole upper body and hair and, to top it all, your sheets completely soaked? Then you know what I am talking about.

I have experienced this a few times and it's very strange. For me it occurred mostly at night, but sometimes also during the day. To begin with, it mostly struck just before my period, but then it started happening all the time. Before I understood what it was, I feared that I had a serious illness. I can advise you not to google night sweats – all sorts of information will come up. I have said it before and I will say it again as a reminder: stop googling! It will only make you more confused. When my best friend told me that during her period she had something verging on bouts of fever once a month, I knew exactly what it was. It wasn't a fever, it was hot flushes!

Having hot flushes is quite normal during the perimenopause. It's estimated that 70 to 75 per cent of all women experience hot flushes, and it's the most common symptom that women seek medical help for. During the perimenopause hot flushes can appear for a while, only to suddenly disappear and come back later on. As with everything else, there is no one rule for everybody; instead, the frequency and degree are completely individual. For some women, the hot flushes don't appear until they are very near the menopause; for others they continue way after their last period.

A hot flush can range from a mild warmth in your body to the unpleasant sensation that a bucket of warm juice has been poured over you. Warm, wet and sticky, with a topping of something that is akin to anxiety. The way most people describe the classic hot flush is the feeling of heat over your face, shoulders, head and upper body. You often sense in advance that a hot flush is imminent. You can feel worried or anxious, or just that something is wrong with your body.

What happens during a hot flush is that the body heats up, just like when you have a fever or exercise hard. A study with sensors has shown that the body's outer temperature can rise by up to four degrees during a hot flush. The blood flow increases, which makes the skin hot and flushing. The body's reaction to this acute rise in temperature is to try to cool down. The same system that kicks in during a fever is triggered here too, and for many women this means an attack of extreme sweating. Some start to shiver despite being sweaty and some don't sweat at all. And then there are the unfortunate women who experience a hot sweat and a cold sweat at the same time.

Some women experience other vasomotor problems during this period. These can manifest themselves as palpitations, irregular heartbeat or a racing heart; it seems like anything and everything can occur during the perimenopause. I suffered particularly from strange heart rhythms, which was a very unpleasant experience. I have had arrhythmia – disrupted heart rhythm – for a very long time, which I have luckily been able to keep in check with medication. During the perimenopause it worsened acutely, and I had to increase my dose.

Hot flushes are not something that's made up. Far from

it. They can be a very unpleasant experience and I even believe they can be confused with a panic attack or a fall in blood pressure if they occur during the day. I have been lucky enough to experience hot flushes mainly at night. But some women can feel dizzy, as if they have had a sudden drop in blood pressure.

Hot flushes can last for anything from a few seconds to a couple of minutes, and may occur once during the night or fifty times during the day. So, as I said, it's very individual, but researchers have still been able to find a few commonalities. For example, hot flushes often appear between one o'clock and three o'clock at night; some studies suggest this may be because oestrogen levels are naturally lowest at night. Many women lie awake during these hours, which could be because of the hot flushes. It's also hard to say at which age hot flushes begin. But what seems to be common is that they sneak up on you at the start of the perimenopause, and then occur more often as you get closer to the menopause.

There may also be a connection between more hot flushes and being overweight, smoking, alcohol, sleeplessness, caffeine, stress and eating too many carbohydrates. Scientists, however, are not completely agreed on the causes, and it's hard to tell if you have more hot flushes because you're overweight or because of other factors in your lifestyle. Several studies have, on the other hand, shown that smoking can affect your symptoms during the perimeno-pause, so giving up smoking is a good first step. I also have friends who have given up coffee and alcohol and whose hot flushes have lessened or even stopped altogether.

Hot flushes and sleeplessness are closely linked, but it's not always the hot flushes that cause the sleeplessness. It is, however, safe to say that the aftermath (sweating) of a hot flush *always* wakes you up. In other words, one thing leads to another. At the same time, some of us don't get hot flushes; instead we just can't sleep and feel low.

## Insomnia

As I have said, what I found the worst to endure was the inability to sleep, and for me this was partly caused by hot flushes. It's no myth that a lack of sleep can drive you mad, even though the media sometimes try to make out that people can power through life with very little sleep. There is even a term for this that I have encountered in many international health publications: the sleepless elite – as if not sleeping were a merit.

But it's not good not to sleep. Having a good sleep pattern is essential. Not just because a lack of sleep can lead to poor mental health, but also because it's dangerous from a physiological perspective. Sleep is required by the body and the brain to recover and process experiences. The need for sleep differs between different people, but it is generally accepted that a grown adult should have between six and nine hours of sleep to be well rested. Scientists from Oxford, Cambridge and Harvard universities have concluded that, on average, we sleep two hours less today than we did in the 1960s and that, as a consequence, our health has suffered. One scientist even claimed that a lack of sleep is as bad for our health as the overconsumption of sugar, and can be seen as the next big health hazard of our time.

During sleep, a growth hormone is released that helps insulin to store sugar. If this is disrupted, the storage of the sugar doesn't work that well. After just a couple of days, too much sugar will be circulating in your blood and after a week you will have levels that can be comparable to those of a diabetic. Diabetes is an illness that can also ultimately affect your heart. So if you raise the risk of diabetes, the risk of heart and vascular disease also increases. When you stop sleeping properly you are also more prone to depression and burnout, both of which are reactions to long-term stress; lack of sleep is enormously stressful for your body.

How long can you cope without sleeping? A rat can go without sleep for four to five weeks before it dies. Far less time is needed for you to become a zombie. Nobody really knows how long a human being can go without sleep before they die, but the holder of the Guinness World Record for being awake for the longest time is a seventeen-year-old student who did not sleep for 264 hours. For eleven days he was completely awake. After that he slept for just over fourteen hours and appeared completely restored. This is, however, not something I recommend you try!

There are two hormones above all that affect sleep. One is cortisol, which is a stress and alertness hormone, and the other is melatonin – our sleep hormone. We are all programmed with a daily bodily rhythm known as a circadian rhythm, which is about twenty-four hours long – as long as a day. The circadian rhythm affects the production of both cortisol and melatonin.

The daily rhythm is regulated by an interaction in your brain, and the body's manufacturing of melatonin is stimulated by darkness. This makes you sleep better when it's dark, and normally you don't have a problem staying awake when it's light outside. For a healthy person, cortisol peaks in the morning and before lunch, when you most need energy to get going. Then cortisol decreases throughout the day, to be at its lowest level in the evening and at night when you are preparing for sleep. Melatonin is a sleep hormone that makes you feel tired; it helps you to go to sleep and remain asleep throughout the night. The level of melatonin is at its highest during the evening and at night.

When you enter the perimenopause and your hormones

start to change, your stress and sleep hormones are affected too. Some people suffer from reduced cortisol levels and find it difficult to get up in the morning. Some experience an energy dip at two or three o'clock in the afternoon. Others have too little melatonin when going to sleep.

Levels of cortisol and melatonin change during the perimenopause, and with age (and possibly raised stress levels) melatonin decreases in both men and women. Too little melatonin prevents us from going into a deep sleep, with the result that we never feel truly well rested. Moreover, sleep deprivation can lead to many other symptoms, so let me tell you this: sleep is the first thing you need to fix – then all other problems will be easier to handle.

## Feeling over-emotional

I hope that you now have a slightly better understanding of why you may be sleepless and sweaty. But let's get to perhaps the most important part – why do you feel down? This affects us most of all. To walk around every day and not feel calm, harmonious and happy but instead down, sad and low is really hard. You may be irritated and angry. You may cry and have panic attacks. Or perhaps you wake in the middle of the night feeling paranoid. You have strange thoughts about terrible things that could happen, like someone dying or becoming ill. Or you may become anxious that someone at work is trying to steal your position. These thoughts often have no bearing on reality whatsoever.

I will never forget the first time I woke up with heart palpitations. It was very unpleasant, and at night everything always feels extra-difficult. I lay in the darkness thinking that if I fell asleep I may never wake up again. What if I was having a heart attack?

The thoughts that pop up in the early hours of the morning can be a little intense, and that in itself is nothing strange or unusual. But it's good to be aware that hormonal changes during the perimenopause also affect our feel-good hormones and that this can become a vicious circle, for when the feel-good hormone serotonin decreases our sleep is affected. In other words, fluctuating hormones lead to changes in serotonin levels, which can result in poor sleep. So it's understandable that we feel low and have problems sleeping. A lack of serotonin can also bring on depression. All these hormones seem to affect one another, and therefore the entire system is disrupted.

**REDUCED OESTROGEN/
PROGESTERONE**

Leads to decreased
serotonin and problems
with melatonin.

Leads to hot flushes.

**YOU GET SLEEPLESS,
SWEATY, AND LOW**

*Sleep cycle with reduced oestrogen/progesterone*

As you can see, sleep plays a central part in your overall well-being. It is important that you deal with any issues before they make you feel worse. It's also important to investigate any sleep problems to ensure they aren't a sign of something else. In some cases, solving your sleep problems may be enough to fix your fluctuating hormones.

Don't despair. There is always something you can do to feel better. Your perimenopower is with you.

## Symptoms

anxiety

depression

dry mucus membranes

frequent need to urinate

headaches

heart palpitations

hot flushes/flashes

insomnia

irregular periods

joint and muscle pain

mood swings

night sweats

panic attacks

reduced sex drive

spotting

tiredness

unusually heavy bleeding

weight gain

# 6

# Don't Panic

'Exercise is a good drug. Become addicted to it and you'll feel better, you'll see.'

**A TEXT MESSAGE FROM ONE
OF MY DOCTOR FRIENDS**

If you feel the same as I did, that you will try *anything* not to have these strange symptoms, you have come to the right place, for I have some good news. The first, and possibly most important, thing you can do to relieve the hormonal unease in your body is to take care of it from the inside out. I am sure you've read masses about miracle diets and training programmes to get into top physical shape, perhaps with the main purpose of conforming to the norm of how you 'should' look. But the fact is that exercise and the right diet, more than anything else, will make you *feel better*, even during the perimenopause. It's not exactly rocket science, but it's good to be reminded every now and then about why you need to look after your body.

## Dare to try something new

For a long time after my hormones started to go haywire, I found it hard to pull myself together. I was both worried and frustrated about all the strange things that were happening, and the last thing I wanted to do was to go out jogging. It would feel so much better to sit on the couch with my hand reaching into a packet of crisps instead. Do you recognise this in yourself?

But maybe it's time to try something new. Regardless of how well you look after your body already, you might feel better if you change something in your lifestyle. After all, everything in life is connected, and even though our mental well-being is largely influenced by external factors like the weather, our finances and our relationships with our boss, partner or parents, it's amazing how much we can affect our bodies with the help of what we put in our mouths and how much we exercise.

All our symptoms are also connected. If you have night sweats, it affects your sleep. If you sleep badly, you feel low. If you are low, it can be hard to look after yourself properly. But breaking the downward spiral is easier than you think, if you know what to do.

## Small changes make a big difference

In Part Two – Help Is at Hand – you will learn what I did to lessen my problems. Yes, your guess is right: food and exercise. During the first years of my perimenopause, I realised that these were my saviours: food and exercise were the remedies that had the greatest influence on how I felt. After all, the body is a machine and if we look after it correctly with regular sleep, healthy food and physical activity, it will continue to work optimally, even during the perimenopause.

Now don't misunderstand me: I don't mean that you necessarily have to make a complete change and become a fitness fanatic living solely on vegetable smoothies (though if you choose to go all in with that lifestyle, go for it!). What I want to say is that, regardless of where in life you are right now, you may witness miracles just by taking an extra walk every so often. A power walk is a great recipe for kick-starting your perimenopower!

By changing your lifestyle, you can provide your body with the best conditions for regaining its balance. But if that's not enough for you, I have a few aces up my sleeve further on in the book. You see, I want you to know *everything*, absolutely everything, to work out how you can get help. I want to reassure you that sooner or later you will find the balance that works wonders for you and you won't have to wake up sweaty and confused at night.

If you look upon this period as a time in your life when you will give yourself more consideration and attention than ever before, then you are on the right road to finding your perimenopower. More care and more love towards yourself are the first things you need during the initial years when the hormones begin to change. If you give yourself the best conditions, the transition will be easier for you. I believe you are just like me. You just want the bad stuff to go away and to feel like yourself again.

I want to congratulate you for coming to the right place to reclaim the power that is in you. In the following chapters, I will show you which keys I used to unlock my perimenopower. I knew it was there – I just hadn't seen it for a very long time.

**Loss of Confidence:** many women find they lose their confidence over things they had previously taken for granted, such as driving a car or travelling alone. This loss of confidence is caused by a drop in oestrogen, which can lead to the adrenal glands going into overdrive, increasing worry and anxiety. HRT may be helpful, as are therapy and mindfulness techniques such as meditation.

# PART TWO

## Help Is at Hand

# 7

# Sleep Like a Queen

'Sleep had always been my superpower –
even raising three children I could always
get a decent night's rest. But when I hit my
mid-forties, suddenly I was lying awake half
the night.'

**CLAIRE, FORTY-SIX**

The root of much of the evil in the perimenopause is disturbed sleep. I'd go as far as to say it's the root of all evil. Insomnia isn't something you can ignore or push aside, it affects *your entire existence*.

When I had my first bouts of sleeplessness and started talking about what I was going through, it became apparent that many of my friends struggled with similar problems. One of them told me that she always woke up at around two or three o'clock at night and couldn't get back to sleep, so she simply got up and baked instead. She never slept for more than five hours, not even at weekends. She is one of those people who claims not to need a lot of sleep and is able to function anyway. My answer to that is usually that it's a myth that you can cope without sleeping in the long term.

Another friend told me that she never fell into a deep sleep since she woke up every time her husband rolled over. She slept so lightly that she never felt rested. Several others also told me they sweated so much during the night that they had to get up and take a shower. And then there is the poor friend who didn't sleep for two weeks and was admitted to a psychiatric unit; now she needs to take a small white pill every night to be able to sleep so that she can function at all. She will probably have to do this for many years to come.

The human body is designed to sleep at night. In the same way that you must charge your cell phone regularly, you too need to be 'charged' with new energy overnight. And five hours isn't enough, end of story. How are your sleep patterns? And have they changed lately? Do you often wake up at night, and does it take some time before you can get back to sleep? Are you sweating more than normal but haven't considered getting help for it?

One way to minimise the risk of waking up sweating in the middle of the night is to have a nice, cool bedroom and a duvet that's not too warm. If that doesn't work, use my tips below, and if none of those help you should, of course, seek medical advice.

## Everything starts with a good night's sleep

Perhaps, before the perimenopause, on a normal night you would fall asleep just like that – bam! – and then wake up – bam! – completely rested and feeling amazing. But these days I have learned that it's a little more complicated to achieve a full night's rest.

Over the course of a normal night, we sleep in several consecutive sleep cycles. Each cycle lasts for around an hour and a half, and throughout the cycle we sleep both deeply and lightly. When the sleep cycle is finished, we wake up for a few seconds before the next one starts, but we hardly ever remember this. It may sound strange, since we don't recall the micro-awakening, but it's true. I have been told that you need to be awake for up to five minutes to be able to remember it afterwards.

But, despite sleeping more lightly at times throughout the night, we are not intended to wake up regularly just because our partner snores or rolls over. We shouldn't have to change sheets in the middle of the night either. If you constantly wake up, you will never enter the deep-sleep state that the body needs to recover properly. Luckily, help is at hand. I have tried everything, and I would like to share what I have found to be useful. Hopefully something will work for you too.

## 1. <u>Avoid caffeine</u>

I undoubtedly slept my best when I stopped drinking coffee altogether. Caffeine has a stimulating effect on the body, and therefore a complete break from it can make a huge difference in the way you feel and, above all, how you sleep. If you, like many others, find it hard to function normally without your morning coffee, consider letting the first cup of the day also be your last. Try it for a week and see if you experience any difference in how well you sleep.

## 2. <u>Exercise</u>

Exercise increases your feel-good endorphins and can help you sleep better. When I exercise regularly, it becomes very obvious that I sleep better than when I exercise less. My brain is no longer in overdrive, because I feel that when my body is tired, my brain doesn't have the energy to cause me any trouble. On the other hand, during periods when I haven't exercised, I have felt as though my thoughts are like an old scratched record. I lie in bed thinking so much that I can't relax and then I can't sleep at all.

I have noticed, though, that exercising too close to

bedtime is not to be recommended. When you exercise, your body gets energised before it can start to relax, so you will need sufficient time to unwind. I try to avoid exercising after eight o'clock at night, which works well for me.

## 3. <u>Yoga</u>

Start a beginner's course or look for yoga instructions online. Do a couple of yoga exercises at home every day for a month – fifteen minutes at a time is enough. I promise that you will start sleeping better. But perhaps you have already tried yoga and feel that it's not your cup of tea. Maybe you are like a friend of mine, who glared at me and said: 'Katarina, if you tell me one more time to start yoga so I can sleep again, I'm going to end our friendship.' We laughed and realised that she was probably not in the right headspace for yoga. I completely understand that – not everyone wants to do yoga and many people feel it's far too slow. But the fact is, yoga makes the body relax, and in my case it felt as though yoga pulled me out of the state of tension I was in.

There is a particular type of yoga which I found incredibly useful for improving my sleep. I even used to call it sleep yoga. Every Friday, I went to a class called Restorative Yoga. The idea was that you would lie in relaxing positions for a very long time with the help of bolsters, cushions and warm blankets. It wasn't about getting sweaty or doing handstands. It was about relaxation – the deepest kind of relaxation you could ever imagine. I can't even describe what went on during those ninety minutes. During some classes, I felt as if I was somewhere between being asleep and awake. You can find this kind of class at many studios – it's often called Yin Yoga, Restorative Yoga or Yoga Nidra (which is just the relaxation part, with no physical exercises).

After a class like that I was incredibly relaxed, but at the same time I felt as if I had an extreme regeneration of energy. I was rested yet at the same time so alert. During my terrible period of insomnia, I knew that I would sleep better at the weekend if I went to my sleep yoga. After those classes I had at least two sleep-filled nights in a row.

Yoga helped me, and I hope that, even if you are not there yet, one day you will get into the yoga headspace.

## 4. Acupressure mat

The acupressure mat is a relaxing product originating from yoga. It is a mat with hundreds of tiny spikes, whose only function is that you should lie on it. I understand if you think it sounds strange – I did too. But acupressure mats have been used by people who practise yoga for many years, and when one of my close friends started to rave about hers, I decided to try it.

Just as you might imagine, lying down on a bed of tiny nails hurts a little at first. But it also gets your blood circulation going and, in a strange way, it calms your body down. The mat has a relaxing effect, particularly during times of stress.

At one stage, I would lie down on my mat in bed at night and fall asleep on it. Although it was uncomfortable, it was as if the pain made the body focus on relaxing. In the end, I would fall asleep. During my worst periods of sleeplessness, I even brought my mat with me in my suitcase so that I could sleep better when I was away.

The acupressure mat is said to generate a state of deep relaxation and it worked for me. Sure, I would wake up to remove the mat at some point in the night, but I often went straight back to sleep. And if I woke in the middle of the night I would sometimes get it out again because I knew it worked.

## 5. Evening bath

Another thing that I made a habit of when I couldn't sleep was to run a bath. I lit scented candles, added some lavender oil and floated in darkness for half an hour. To combine warmth and water, like in the uterus, pleasantly relaxes your body, and lavender oil has a beneficial effect in calming your senses. On many occasions I have fallen fast asleep afterwards. If you like going to a spa, you will know exactly what I mean. Sometimes a calm and warm environment is all your body needs to let go of the tension, relax and fall asleep.

I hope you will sleep better after trying my tips. Wouldn't it be wonderful to discover that, as long as you are kind to your body, allowing it to unwind, you will become friends with it? For this is what it feels like when you are right in the middle of your worst phase: as if you have fallen out with your own body and you are prepared to do anything to become friends again.

During the first years of the perimenopause, when the hormones first began to fight each other, the things I've mentioned above were enough for me to become calmer. But the closer I got to menopause the more insistent my troubles became, and I entered the world of supplements and unprescribed medication.

I would like to tell you about the ones that I personally found most useful, but I want to make it clear that I am not a doctor and that the medication that worked for me may not work as well for you and your body. Nothing beats the personal advice and care provided by your medical centre or gynaecologist. My aim isn't to recommend these supplements, it's just to introduce you to a few of those that are available so that you will *know there is help* and that sometimes that help is packaged in small jars or plastic strips. There is nothing wrong in giving your body the help it needs. Many of the medicines we use are meant to mimic as closely as possible the vitamins, hormones or other substances we have naturally in our bodies but which, for some reason, we need more of.

I also want to make the point that I am not an advocate of stuffing my body full of medicine, as I am sure you have already understood. I am completely convinced that the biggest changes come from our lifestyle, the sort of things I mentioned in sections 1 to 5 above. Sections 6 to 8 below are aimed at those who have more severe problems and for whom none of the above provide sufficient effect.

## 6. <u>Natural supplements</u>

Health food stores sell natural supplements that have a calming effect and may help you to start sleeping again. One example is *valerian*. It's a perennial herb that grows in both Europe and Asia. Another natural remedy with a calming effect is a trendy newcomer in the health food business, the herb *ashwagandha*. Both valerian and ashwagandha are calming and are used to treat anxiety. Many people take valerian in order to sleep or to relax, and if your sleep problems are moderate, valerian can help. I used valerian during the day for a while and didn't feel as wound-up. Ashwagandha is said to have the same effect, but I myself haven't tried it for long enough to notice any significant difference to my sleep.

## 7. Melatonin

Another medicine, or rather hormone, that I would like to mention is melatonin. Melatonin is the hormone that's most important for our sleep. We produce it naturally and it makes our bodies understand when it's day and when it's night. With age, the production of melatonin decreases, and it can also decrease during periods of severe stress. If you have other hormone problems, the level decreases even further. If the level decreases beyond the optimum you will have trouble sleeping; moreover, melatonin has also been shown to be important to our feel-good hormones. Just like the sex hormone oestrogen.

So, if both melatonin and oestrogen decrease, the inevitable result is that you have trouble sleeping. And if that also affects our feel-good hormone, serotonin, we sleep badly *and* we feel down. Of course, it's difficult to know if you are feeling low because you are sleeping badly or if you are sleeping badly because you are feeling low. So it's not just a restless mind and hot flushes that cause sleep problems: it can also be because your level of sleep hormones has been disrupted.

In August 2017, a major British meta-analysis was conducted in which a research team compared 5,030 studies to determine if conclusions could be drawn on the real effects of melatonin – in other words, if melatonin as a supplement was effective against sleeplessness. It showed that melatonin has a clear effect on those who can't sleep compared to placebo patients (who *thought* they had taken the medicine but had actually just taken a sugar pill).

In Europe and the United States, melatonin is sold like any other vitamin, while in other countries, such as the UK and Sweden, it's still subject to much debate. It's argued that just because it's natural, it doesn't mean it's good. This, of course, is true – not everything natural is necessarily good for you. But it's interesting that views on melatonin differ so much throughout the world, and that some countries are more restrictive than others.

I spoke to Professor Torbjörn Åkerstedt, who is part of a research group focusing on stress, sleep and recovery, and he had many interesting things to say about sleeping and melatonin. When I asked him why he didn't think melatonin is that popular as a medicine in some parts of the world, he answered that the reason might be because melatonin is natural and therefore it can't be patented. In other words, there is no money for research or profit, so few people will want to invest money in producing it. Torbjörn also mentioned research that shows that melatonin is not just good for your sleep but is also proven to have anti-cancer effects that counteract mutations in the cells. On the other hand, there are studies which indicate that melatonin is more or less without side effects, good or bad.

As I have mentioned, our natural melatonin production decreases with age, and if exercise, restorative yoga and natural remedies don't help you sleep better, melatonin may be an option. If it proves to give you other health benefits as well, that's just a bonus. It's not without reason that melatonin is known as a miracle drug in the United States.

## 8. Atarax

Once I started to sleep better, I still felt anxious now and again. So I asked my gynaecologist if she could suggest something that would help with anxiety and make me relax. For even if I could sleep, my body sometimes felt tense, as though I was unable to wind down. Have you ever felt like that?

I was clear that I wanted to avoid antidepressants, sleeping pills and anxiety suppressants. I asked for an alternative that was not addictive but could just be taken now and then. She suggested I try Atarax. Even though, as I have said, I am very dubious about using medication if it can be avoided, I would like to tell you about how Atarax worked for me and why I tried it at all.

Atarax is an antihistamine given, for example, to small children to ease the itching of chickenpox. It blocks histamine, a substance that can sometimes cause allergic reactions in certain cells. Atarax has also been shown to work against anxiety and worry, since it makes your muscles relax, but it has no proven effect on sleeping problems. It's also not addictive. For me, Atarax is so relaxing that I fall asleep after taking the smallest dose of ten milligrams. I have taken it when I felt uneasy and worried, and sometimes if I have slept badly for two nights in a row. On the third night I will take Atarax finally to get a good night's sleep. When things were at their worst for me, having melatonin and Atarax to hand was a great comfort.

## Do the easiest things first

Now I have given you eight tips on how to improve your sleep; I believe and hope that they will really make a difference for you. At the very least they should help you to get a good night's sleep every so often. For now, maybe you only need to follow these tips for a couple of days per month. Maybe you sleep well except during ovulation and during your period. Maybe the menopause is still a long way ahead of you. As it comes closer, sleep problems may appear at any time during your cycle, not just during ovulation and your period. And then it's important to look after yourself in every way that you can.

I recommend you try these tips in order. If your sleeping problems are severe, you may not find a solution until you are way down the list. If your sleep problems are infrequent, you might manage by using the first few tips. Anyway – off you go and sleep well!

# Katarina's sleep solutions

1. Avoid caffeine

2. Exercise

3. Yoga

4. Acupressure mat

5. Evening bath

6. Natural supplements

7. Melatonin

8. Atarax

# 8

# Get in the Mood
# with Food

'Let food be thy medicine and medicine
be thy food.'

**HIPPOCRATES**

Recent scientific research has proven to us what Hippocrates knew thousands of years ago – that food can change how you feel. Masses of scientific studies on diet are being conducted, countless books are being written, and the number of health coaches and bloggers focusing on healthy food grows every year.

I recently read about a Japanese professor who was 105 years old. His advice for a long life was that you should 'worry less about eating healthily'. This is interesting because the worry about eating healthily enough is, in itself, unhealthy and can lead to expectations that are hard to live up to. But I still feel that if you are ever going to attempt to eat more healthily, it's during this period of your life that you should be trying to take extra care of yourself. As I have said, this is a phase when many things are happening within your body, and if you realise this and give your body the right type of 'fuel' it will work the way you want it to. When you are aware of the impact that food has on your perimenopausal systems, you can begin to use it to feel better.

## Food has a greater effect than you think

Sometimes I feel there are so many new findings on health foods that I can hardly keep track of them. It's not always easy knowing what is best for you; some experts say that food plays an extremely important role in your overall health, while others say it doesn't matter as much as you think. But there are several studies that indicate that food may have a significant effect in regulating perimenopausal symptoms.

Asian women, for example, report far fewer problems with hot flushes than Western women. Theories as to why this happens vary, but many believe the reason to be the Asians' enormous consumption of soy. Soy contains phytoestrogen – a plant material similar to the oestrogen produced naturally in the body; so the phytoestrogens in soy may have an effect on the likelihood of suffering hot flushes. But the phytoestrogen in soy is so weak that it would take a complete change in diet for us Westerners to be able to benefit from it. In other words, a whole lot of tofu. But it's still interesting that diet can affect the symptoms so significantly.

Another food category that has a bearing on health is spicy food. Sometimes when I eat spicy food I begin to sweat – the heat in my mouth seems to affect the rest of my body too. Does this sound familiar? Since one of our most common symptoms during the perimenopause is sweating, it might be a good idea to avoid hot, spicy food if this is a particular problem for you. Some women report that spicy food is a trigger for a hot flush.

It's also interesting to see a connection between health and meat consumption. There have been several studies over the past few years showing that a plant-based diet is healthier than a meat-based one. The World Health Organization has even distributed a warning that processed meat products can be as dangerous to your health as smoking. It may seem strange that a food which most of us eat every day can be so harmful. But there may be something to it.

An American study with over 90,000 respondents showed that vegetarian diets led to a decreased risk of heart and vascular diseases, high blood pressure, type 2 diabetes and some forms of cancer. A British study with over 65,000 respondents had the same result. Conversely, the risks increased when regularly eating large amounts of meat. Yet it's still very difficult for many of us to switch the beef casserole to a vegetarian equivalent.

I never used to pay much attention to what I ate on a day-to-day basis. I was often under a lot of stress and worked long hours and constantly felt guilty about the children. I always made sure they got lots of good, nutritious food, but I neglected myself. Frequently, I didn't have time for breakfast and instead ate something in front of my computer. There were many quick carbohydrate snacks and I could go for long periods without thinking about what I put in my mouth. But somewhere in the back of my head, I started to wonder how my future health was going to be affected by what I did to my body.

I love food and see it as one of the great pleasures in life. I enjoy going to good restaurants and one of my favourite meals is steak tartare. But I don't eat steak tartare every day. When it comes to food I believe in moderation. I fully respect all types of diet and food preferences, but I believe that a balanced diet is what the body needs. So this chapter is about the kinds of food that helped me to feel better during my perimenopause.

## Cut down on meat

When I heard about the positive effects vegetarian food has on your health, I decided to eat solely vegetarian food for a few weeks. I wanted to find out if the claims about meat were right.

I measured my cholesterol levels before I started, ate vegetarian food for three months (I'll be honest and confess to cheating a few times with salmon), and measured my cholesterol levels again afterwards. Although my levels were good before the diet change, they were even better after I stopped eating meat. I also noticed that my perimenopausal symptoms had decreased. I rarely suffered night sweats and, when I did, it was only during my period. Nowadays I eat a little meat again. I rarely cook it at home, but if I am invited out and beef casserole is served, I will have it.

## Limit sugar and simple carbohydrates

I strived to live a healthy lifestyle and tried to avoid junk food with a lot of fat and sugar, and I noticed that, with these small changes, my symptoms decreased. Before, it was as if I had a problem with my blood sugar. It went up and down along with my mood. Now I don't sense these variations any more. Blood sugar levels are more stable when you don't eat food rich in sugar or carbohydrates. Many women have blood sugar problems during this period without having diabetes, and I was one of them. If I didn't eat every three hours I was shaky. I also felt extremely tired after each meal, as if eating drained me of energy in a way that it hadn't before.

All of this is connected to sex-hormone changes. When there is a dispute in the sex-hormone camp, other hormones are also affected. There is research being conducted today on what happens to your body during this time, but what is known is that changes in oestrogen indirectly affect blood sugar.

Letting go of sugar was really hard for me, but I had to do it. I was not feeling good because of my large sugar intake, which came mainly in the form of eating sweets, chocolate and ice cream several times a week. But when I cut down on white sugar I felt a significant difference. I haven't been picky about the 'hidden' sugar, for example in ketchup, muesli, bread and so on, but I have tried cutting out sweets at least during the week.

Of course, it's important to have carbohydrates, but try to choose the so-called slow-release ones that take longer for the body to absorb into the blood and don't create the quick 'sugar rush' that comes from carbohydrates found in ice cream, sweets, bread and pasta. Slow carbohydrates, however, give a longer feeling of fullness and are found in, among other things, beans, brown pasta and brown rice.

## Don't give up!

At the time when I was feeling at my worst and having problems sleeping, I found it very hard to think about eating healthily. My body was in overdrive and I sometimes felt that I could hardly keep my head above water. All I wanted was to eat junk food, skip exercise and just go to bed.

When you are not sleeping, your body is under extreme stress; you are tired, yet your body is hyper. The less you sleep, the higher the level of stress, which in turn leads to a larger appetite. Did you know that many people eat junk food when they are stressed out? This is partly because they lack the energy to cook healthy food and partly because the body is crying out for quick energy, which you get from junk food. No wonder my body was craving fast carbohydrates which would give me energy when I hadn't slept.

I also noticed that, when I slept and ate badly, I slowly but surely started to gain weight. Even when I exercised and ate as I had always done, I put on weight. I thought that this was odd until I learned that, during the perimenopause, your metabolism slows down, making it easier to put on the pounds. So don't worry if you suddenly start gaining weight without having made any major changes to your lifestyle – it's completely normal. But it's yet another reason to think about whether you need to change something in your daily routine to compensate for your decreased metabolism. Maybe you can manage on smaller portions than before, since you are using less energy?

A consequence of weight gain can be an increase in perimenopausal problems. Some studies have shown that those with high cholesterol (which is often connected with being overweight) often suffer more from hot flushes and sweating than others. If you, like me, start eating more plant-based food, your cholesterol levels can improve and you may experience fewer problems. If you care about what goes on in your body and put your mind to it, you will at least minimise the risk of problems. Once I understood the connection between food, sleep and weight, it inspired me to be kind to my body in order to set things right.

## Limit caffeine and alcohol

I also noticed other symptoms directly connected to my diet. For example, I experienced palpitations when I drank too much coffee or alcohol, which I had never experienced before. My body told me clearly that something wasn't right. I hadn't been listening to it, but now it was time to do so. I concluded that if I exercised more and ate better I would find my superpower again. So I tried to do everything I could to navigate my way through the different diets and theories.

## Try the Mediterranean diet

My conclusion, having read numerous studies, articles, books and blogs, and based on the results of my own experience, is that the diet with the best effect on perimenopausal symptoms is the so-called Mediterranean one. It's a balanced way of eating that isn't so much about what you cut out as about eating a little of everything and, above all, things that provide long-term energy rather than quick energy. You even eat red meat with the Mediterranean diet, but far less of it. It contains a lot of fruit and vegetables, nuts, pulses, vegetable oils, whole grains and fish, and less red meat, milk and dairy produce.

Hamburgers, french fries, sausages, sweets and ice cream are a few examples of what we call junk food. How do you feel when you have had salmon and salad compared to when you have eaten a burger with bread and dressing? If you cut out junk food the fat storage within your body decreases, and if you add healthy greens and a lot of protein you will feel much better.

## Do you need supplements?

Minor changes here and there can do a lot of all-round good. My advice is for your diet to contain mainly protein, fibre, fruit and vegetables and healthy fats such as nuts, avocado and olive oil. Be careful with carbohydrates and dairy produce. Nowadays most of these can be replaced with, for example, soy and oat products. Avoid sugar and cut down on meat (especially red meat) and junk food such as processed foods and fast food. If you don't get enough vitamins from your food, you may need to think about supplements.

Some doctors say that you don't need to take supplements

unless you have any deficiencies – in other words, illnesses brought about by abnormally low levels of vitamins or other essentials that your body really needs. However, vegans are recommended to take an extra supplement of iron and vitamin B12 as these can be difficult to obtain from a completely vegan diet. There are also those who recommend a supplement of omega 3 if, for example, you don't eat fish.

Personally, I have used supplements at certain times. For example, at one stage I often had infections in my body and so I took extra vitamin C. In Sweden we have many dark months and therefore it may be a good idea to take additional vitamin D to compensate for the lack of sun.

During the perimenopause, I have also chosen to help my body by taking a few more supplements. My gynaecologist recommended that I take vitamin B, especially B6. Vitamin B6 is needed for the brain cells to function normally, and a lack of vitamin B can cause you to feel low and irritated. A lack of vitamin B12 can even increase the risk of depression. Therefore taking vitamin B can make you feel less down during the perimenopause.

I also take supplements of magnesium, a mineral. A lack of magnesium can, as well as having some physical symptoms, also cause psychological problems such as depression or mental tiredness. Several dieticians claim that you sleep better if you take magnesium, and since this has been my biggest problem, I choose to take it.

My own experiences tell me that Hippocrates may have been right. What if food can be our medicine? It's the simplest and most accessible way to change how we feel.

**B6** is found mainly in animal-based food, but also in potatoes, grains and berries. Among other things, it is very important for the functioning of the nerves.

**B12** is plentiful in animal-based products. Fish, meat and shellfish, for example, contain high levels of **B12**. Vegans are recommended to take a supplement of **B12** as it's an important vitamin that you should not be deficient in. It is needed for metabolism within the cells and the production of blood cells but is also said to have an important function for the nervous system.

**Vitamin C** is perhaps the best-known vitamin, the one that everyone talks about. It's an antioxidant that, among other things, helps to keep us healthy. It's found in most vegetables, berries and fruits.

**Vitamin D** is needed for strong bones, teeth and the immune system. It also affects our mood. We obtain it in two ways: from the sun and from certain foods such as fish, dairy products and eggs.

**Iron.** Among other things, iron is needed to transport oxygen from your lungs to your tissues. There is a lot of iron in meat and offal. There is also plenty of iron in pulses and bananas, and green vegetables such as spinach and broccoli. If you are unsure about whether you consume enough, a simple blood test at your medical centre will measure your iron levels.

**Magnesium** is found in pulses, leafy vegetables, whole grains, meat and fish and is needed for normal nerve and muscle function.

**Weight gain:** hormonal triggers during the perimenopause can increase the likelihood of weight gain, particularly around the abdomen. Excess abdominal weight is linked to an increased risk of type 2 diabetes, heart disease and breathing problems.

# 9

# Training Makes
# You Tougher

'After a spinning session I feel at my best.
It's like all my problems are suddenly blown
away.'

**PERNILLA, FORTY-THREE**

I started to suspect a connection between exercise and the perimenopause when a close friend of mine, who was about to turn forty, suddenly couldn't maintain her weight. She had always exercised and eaten healthily but, without having made any changes, she started to put on weight. Her mental state grew worse and she felt very low. On top of this, she also started having problems with her sleep. What was she doing wrong?

Interestingly, we decided that she was exercising far too often and too intensely. When she started replacing some of her workouts with slower sessions and tweaked her diet she began to lose weight, slept better and felt much more energised. My conclusion was that the problems she had been experiencing were connected to changes in her hormones. The intense training that she had earlier managed without any difficulty now caused her difficulties. In her case, the solution was to train less often and less vigorously.

I am the sort of person who needs to put in maximum effort to find exercising fun. In other words, I love high-intensity interval sessions or long spinning classes that exhaust me completely. I had never even considered that this might be bad for my body. But after my friend began feeling better when she cut down on exercise, I started to think more about how training affects perimenopausal symptoms, and that it might not be a simple case of the more exercise the better.

## Over-exercising can raise stress levels

When exercising, the stress levels in your body temporarily increase. Afterwards they decrease again – and they even go down to a lower level than they were at before exercise. But since you are more sensitive to stress during the perimenopause, it can be more difficult than usual for your body to determine what causes this stress and which 'actions' the brain should take. As stress hormones increase, progesterone and oestrogen levels decrease.

Bearing in mind that these hormones naturally decrease during the perimenopause, perhaps it's not such a good idea to do things that lower the levels even more. Perhaps it's sensible to cancel the marathon if you are at a difficult time hormonally. I want to remind you that everything is individual and, if you feel good about training for a marathon, of course you should continue to do so. But if you have started to sense problems and you exercise a lot, it might be worth trying to reduce the training to see if you notice any difference.

The American magazine *Fitness Journal* featured a compilation of several studies on 'Training Through the Transition', in other words exercising during the perimenopause. In them, many scientists agreed that pulse-raising activity of a medium intensity is better for perimenopausal women than high-intensity activity. The more studies I read, the more I realise that there may be advantages to exercising more gently during the perimenopause, particularly if you have problems with sleep.

Many people believe that exercising makes you exert yourself and therefore tires you out, but it's not just down to that. As I mentioned above, exercising vigorously can increase the stress levels in your body, meaning that it takes longer for your body to relax. If you feel more tired than usual you should slow down. During the perimenopause, when your body is over-strained, what it needs is calm and tranquillity, not more stress. If you already exercise hard, be observant if you feel too high afterwards. If this is the case, you should combine your intensive sessions with gentler ones. If you don't have the energy to exercise, be grateful to yourself every time you do manage it.

During my perimenopause, I noticed that I slept worse if I had done a spinning session late at night. I could not wind down afterwards and felt quite hyper. When I did gentler exercise sessions instead, such as Pilates or light weight training, it was far easier to get to sleep that night.

I want to stress that the best training session is the one that actually happens. It's not my intention to suggest that anyone should give up exercise. But do remember that how much you need to exercise in order to notice a difference in your symptoms is individual. *What* you do is less important than the fact that you do *something* physically active. Some people run marathons a couple of times per year; others are satisfied going to the gym once in a while. Just remember to listen to your body and maybe try something new now and again to see if it makes a difference to how you feel.

## Exercise as medicine

Anders Hansen, chief physician in psychiatry and author of several books, insists that exercising is like a hundred medicines. In his book *Brain Power*, he explains how exercising affects the brain. One of his theses is that, in today's society, we find it hard to eliminate stress, and this means that as individuals we should focus on becoming more stress-resistant. And the best way to do this, according to him, is to do exercise, especially any exercise that raises your pulse. There are parts of the brain that work to slow down stress, and research shows that these parts grow when we exercise.

What Hansen means is that, through exercise, we can change how our brain works and thereby influence our mood and well-being. Isn't it great that we have the power to make such an impact? That makes me, at least, more motivated to get out on the running track. Another thing that exercise does is increase production of one of your body's feel-good hormones – endorphins. The effect is so powerful that, during a time when I exercised a lot, I felt worse when I didn't. Exercising had almost become an addiction.

If exercising can have such a significant influence on your brain and such a positive result in decreasing stress, it's not hard to think one step further: that training has a calming and uplifting effect on what you experience during the perimenopause. I understand that it may be difficult to take in the fact that you should exercise while suffering from all sorts of unpleasant symptoms, when you are simply trying to keep your head above water. But I believe that regular physical activity is one of the best things you can do to feel better at this time, and much research supports this. Since sleeping problems and mood swings are issues that we want to nip in the bud during the perimenopause, it speaks for itself that exercise is exactly what we should be doing.

It has also been shown that exercising helps with hot flushes and sweating. Mats Hammar, Professor Emeritus in Gynaecology and Obstetrics at Linköping University in Sweden, was the first in the world to demonstrate that exercising reduced certain symptoms connected to the menopause, especially hot flushes and sweating. One of his theories is that the 'thermostat' in the brain that regulates body temperature doesn't work properly during the menopause and perimenopause, therefore creating hot flushes and sweating. The thermostat is connected to the level of endorphins in your body, which, as we have seen, decreases as the oestrogen decreases. Because of oestrogen reduction, the thermostat believes the body is too hot and sends out blood to the extremities, which causes a sensation of intense heat. This activates the sweat glands in order to lower the body's temperature. In other words, everything is completely confused.

---

## Oestrogen decreases

1  The endorphins become unsettled and endorphin levels are reduced.
2  This reduction affects the thermostat (which regulates your body temperature). The body thinks it's too hot.
3  The brain activates the sweat glands in order to lower the temperature.
4  The hot flush occurs.

---

Now to the really interesting part. Since the level of endorphins directly affects the thermostat's ability accurately to regulate the body's temperature, perhaps the temperature would be more effectively regulated if the endorphin levels increased. Wouldn't it be great if we could influence the release of endorphins somehow? Luckily, Mats Hammar has already figured it out for us.

Mats's study showed that women who exercised regularly generally had fewer symptoms during the menopause, and he concluded that exercise might very well help, especially when the symptoms are to do with sweating and hot flushes. Among other things, physical activity releases a type of endorphin that contributes to the regulation of body temperature. It's a very interesting study that received much attention since it was the first of its kind.

There are also studies that show that after only 150 minutes per week of low-intensity exercise, many women experience fewer perimenopausal problems. You don't have to exercise more than that to enjoy the positive effects of exercising. For some people, three brisk sixty-minute walks per week may be enough. Others would prefer to do three weight-training sessions instead. During the perimenopause, exercising can work just like your food, becoming your medicine. One hundred and fifty minutes of exercise is less than three out of the 168 hours in the week. If it helps you to overcome your problems and make your daily life easier, surely that can be considered time well invested?

**Brain fog:** during the perimenopause, many women describe being unable to recall the right word at the right time, which damages their confidence at work and in social situations. This can lead to feeling anxious about tackling tasks that they'd normally take in their stride.

# 10

# Think Natural

'It's difficult to know which natural remedies work, since everyone says different things about different products. So who should I trust?'

**SARA, FIFTY-ONE**

Now you know how to sort out your sleep, what to eat and how to exercise in order to feel your best. These are the easiest things you can do to feel better. But if you still have problems after trying my suggestions, I would like you to consider natural, plant-based supplements.

## From nature or the lab – what is best?

You could say that plant-based supplements are midway between food and so-called traditional or Western medicine. Apart from the positive effects that your everyday food can give you, there are health benefits to be found in the form of herbs and plants that have been used over the centuries to cure or ease different ailments. You could look at these plant-based supplements as our 'medicine' before there were laboratories that could chemically concoct a mixture of the exact ingredients needed to cure illnesses. This is why this kind of supplement is sometimes called natural or alternative medicine.

One difference between plant-based supplements and the 'normal' medicine prescribed by doctors is that the effects of the supplements are not always scientifically proven. This is because there have not been as many studies of this type of medicine. But even if there isn't always scientific proof that a specific herb works on certain symptoms, many people find it effective. Could it be worth trying it yourself?

Many people believe plant-based medicines to be better than pharmaceutical ones, perhaps because it feels more natural to use ingredients that grow in nature. But there are also those who are critical of natural health supplements, believing them to be not as 'serious' as other medicines. However, in Germany, for example, the situation is different: there alternative medicine is widely acknowledged as a beneficial complement to traditional medicine. Nonetheless, in many other countries there is still a certain scepticism about natural remedies, even though they are becoming more accepted.

The 'alternative' health business turns over a great deal of money, which suggests that we are moving towards greater acceptance of it. Perhaps we have been too harsh towards medicinal plants that have been used for thousands of years on other continents? Or do we need different types of medicines today from those that nature can offer? Perhaps, in the past, we didn't have as much stress around us as we do today? And, undoubtedly, our ancestors ate a completely different diet with less sugar. There were certainly fewer 'lifestyle' diseases back then, such as stress and burnout, and perhaps it was enough to use plants to stay healthy?

I respect both sides of the argument, and perhaps a combination of the two is the best thing – take the best from both. I advise you to gather the information you need to make the right decision for you. Just like ordinary medicines, natural remedies can have side effects, and it's important to be aware of these. Sometimes they can also work badly or not at all if combined with other medicines that you take. Always make sure that you know what you put into your body, and consult your doctor if you are unsure. It's also important to bear in mind that just because something is natural, it doesn't necessarily mean it's good for you.

## Plants in science

I have tried many natural, plant-based supplements and found some that can help to ease problems during the perimenopause. I have even had training as a health food adviser, so I have a good grasp of which natural remedies are on the market. The ones I would like to suggest to you are those which I have either tried personally or read numerous studies about.

### St John's wort

St John's wort (*Hypericum perforatum*) has been in use as a remedy since medieval times and is used today to treat depression. There are studies showing that it is effective in relieving low moods: a German study in 2008, for example, involving 5,500 patients showed that St John's wort had similar effects on depression as other antidepressant treatments, but with fewer side effects. St John's Wort is, therefore, one of the herbs that can be worth trying during the perimenopause if you are feeling low.

### Valerian

Valerian (*Valeriana officinalis*) is another plant that many women take during the perimenopause. It is commonly used to treat sleep problems, since it has a soporific effect. The effects of valerian are somewhat unclear, but there are a couple of studies that show beneficial results. I have tested valerian; it calmed me down and gave me a nice feeling throughout the day.

### Black cohosh

Black cohosh (*Cimicifuga racemosa*) is a plant that may have some effect on perimenopausal symptoms. It has been used by indigenous populations since the dawn of time to ease 'women's problems'. In Germany, black cohosh has been sold as a remedy for more than forty years, and that's where most of the research has been done. Some studies show that black cohosh has a positive effect while others can't find any particular benefits. According to the former, black cohosh reduces sweating, hot flushes, irritability, depression and sleeping problems. Absolutely everything that we want to find a cure for!

### Monk's pepper

Monk's pepper (*Vitex agnus-castus*) is said to have a balancing effect on PMS and hormonal imbalance. Since the perimenopause is considered to have some symptoms in common with PMS, it may be effective to take at this time.

### Pollen extract

There is another plant that appears in this context, and that's pollen extract. There are a few available products containing pollen extract, but there are no major studies showing that it has any effect on the problems of perimenopause, even though a few smaller studies have shown some benefits.

You will find several products containing these ingredients on the shelves of your local health food store. If you are unsure which products to try, I recommend you consult a health food adviser who can guide you in the right direction. The business of natural remedies can be a jungle, and you may receive different answers from various health food advisers as to what will work for your symptoms. The easiest way to find out what is best for you is to test them yourself.

Just as most doctors favour scientifically based medicine, so health food advisers believe that you should use natural remedies. There is bias on both sides. But just because it's natural, it doesn't mean it's good. Have as critical an approach towards natural remedies as you would towards conventional medicine. I don't believe you should stop a medical treatment without having discussed it first with your doctor, so please don't replace a prescribed drug with a 'natural' one without medical advice.

The most important thing is to have an open mind. There are incredible medicines that we humans have invented in laboratories, just as there are incredible herbs in nature. If you feel that you have found the right path using natural remedies, I would like to congratulate you. The rest of you can stay with me for the next chapter, for now we have arrived at the last option. Perhaps you have been holding on for several years, managing with lifestyle changes and natural remedies and feeling great; but now, as you are getting towards the end of your perimenopause, suddenly you feel that approach isn't working 100 per cent any more. The problems often get worse the closer you get to the menopause. But stay calm, there is still help at hand!

**Headaches:** oestrogen works to dilate blood vessels, while progesterone contracts them. As these hormones fluctuate during the perimenopause, headaches may be experienced more than usual. If you suffer from migraines, they may get worse during the perimenopause.

# 11

# To HRT or Not to HRT

'When I began taking oestrogen, I could feel the difference after just one day. It was as if I had been living in a grey fog, as if my whole existence was muffled. Then it was like waking up from a slow dream and simply becoming normal again.'

**TESS, FORTY-FIVE**

There is probably nothing within women's medicine that is debated more vociferously than the benefits of taking oestrogen. Do you have a friend with breast cancer or an older relative who tells you that oestrogen is dangerous? Or did your mother take oestrogen when you were a teenager? The debate about oestrogen is still confusing to many. In this chapter I would like to straighten out a few questions for you.

## Oestrogen – when nothing else helps

Perhaps you are in a position where you have managed to cope with your perimenopausal symptoms for several years, but feel that things have changed recently. Maybe you've tried everything I have mentioned earlier, such as exercise, changes to your diet, yoga and natural remedies, but they don't help any more. If this is the case, you have probably reached the later phase of the perimenopause when your hormones sink to an extra-low level. Further action may then be needed to solve your problems.

When I reached forty-five, I noticed that certain

symptoms lingered for longer, and I started thinking about whether it was time to begin taking an oestrogen supplement. Then, when I turned forty-eight, I chose to begin using oestrogen patches. These are similar to a plaster, like the kind you would use for a cut or a graze. The patch differs in size depending on the dose, and the idea is that you place it somewhere below your waist. The buttock or thigh is the perfect place. You wear it day and night, which means that oestrogen is released evenly the whole time, and after three to four days you replace it with a new patch.

Just like regular plasters, oestrogen patches are attached with an adhesive that can sometimes cause irritation, especially if your skin is sensitive. This happened to me, so I started using an oestrogen gel instead. The gel is also applied to the lower part of your body: you put a thin layer on an area the size of your palm and leave it to work its way into the skin.

It was my choice to take oestrogen when my perimenopausal problems became too difficult to handle in any other way. But I want to make it clear that just because I chose to do so, it may not be the right thing for you. It's a choice you must make based upon your own symptoms and whether it's worth the possible side effects you may experience.

Like many, I was dubious about taking oestrogen because I had heard of the possible associated risks of breast cancer and heart and vascular disorders. However, after reading masses of studies on the subject and becoming more knowledgeable, I decided to give it a chance. I concluded that the risks were probably not as significant as I had been led to believe, and I considered that the advantages outweighed them.

It was fascinating to see what happened when I started taking oestrogen supplements. The effects were immediate. My skin changed for the better, my hair regained its volume, and above all my ability to sleep returned properly. My mood swings also disappeared, though that may have been due to my sleep being stabilised. My night sweats vanished and there was not a hint of panic attacks or anxiety. All of a sudden, I felt completely rested, glowing and super-happy – the way I had always been deep down. My true personality came back. I really did feel as though I had been given a superpower.

Many of my friends who have taken oestrogen testify to experiencing the same results. For us it was like being born again, or at least being fifteen years younger. But, as with everything else, each of us will react differently to taking these kinds of supplements. Just as some people will feel great exercising vigorously, some will feel fantastic when taking oestrogen, while others will not notice any significant difference.

Please note that if you have had an oestrogen-sensitive breast cancer, current research shows that you should not take oestrogen.

**Hormone Replacement Therapy:**
short- or long-term treatment of
decreasing oestrogen and
progesterone levels.

## Oestrogen must be taken with progesterone

Once you have decided to begin taking oestrogen, you must complement it with a supplement of oestrogen's 'hormone partner', progesterone. These two hormones constitute HRT (Hormone Replacement Therapy), as treatments of combined oestrogen and progesterone are commonly known. The reason why you must also take progesterone is to prevent thickening of the endometrium, which is the inner lining of the uterus. A thickened endometrium is associated with a heightened risk of cancer of the uterus. There is, however, one exception: you don't need to take progesterone if your uterus has been removed, in which case just oestrogen is enough.

Nowadays, oestrogen supplements come in a bioidentical form; previously there was only a synthetic version. Because today's oestrogen is bioidentical, it means that it has the same molecular structure as the body's self-produced hormone. Our body recognises the bioidentical hormone and therefore finds it easier to deal with. You could say that the synthetic version interferes with our body, while the bioidentical one is welcomed by it. It rebalances the body without any greater risk of side effects.

I strongly recommend that the hormones you take are regulated and prescribed. There are alternative ways to get hold of them – from unregulated suppliers – and nowadays you can even buy them on the internet. I cannot recommend that anyone takes hormones without a prescription. And you simply do not know what you are buying online. I believe it is like experimenting with your own body.

Bioidentical oestrogen is available today in the form of tablets, patches, gel and spray. If you take oestrogen through your skin instead of in tablet form, you reduce the possible risks of side effects as the oestrogen doesn't have to pass through the liver as it does when taken as a tablet.

## Attitudes to oestrogen – now and in the past

As little as twenty years ago, it was not unusual for gynaecologists to prescribe oestrogen supplements for menopausal and perimenopausal women. Scientists were unanimous: hormone replacement treatments protected against, among other things, heart and vascular disease. But in 2002, a study was released by the Women's Health Initiative (WHI) which changed the view of oestrogen as a supplement. The study, involving 160,000 women between the ages of fifty and seventy-nine, appeared to show that these treatments could increase the risk of strokes, heart disease and in particular breast cancer. It also reported a heightened risk of ovarian cancer in those who had taken oestrogen.

The study had an enormous impact throughout the world; in Sweden the sale of oestrogen was said to have more than halved immediately. The recommendations on how to take oestrogen were rewritten and the message was that the hormone treatment was only to be prescribed for short periods for acute menopausal problems. The scare was broadcast so loudly and effectively that, even today, women still associate oestrogen with breast cancer. This isn't hard to understand, considering that that we humans have evolved to avoid risks wherever possible. It doesn't always matter how *big* the risks are; that they exist at all is what we focus on.

But times have changed. Lately, there has been growing criticism of the WHI study. Of the thousands of women questioned, the average age was sixty-three and a third of the women were being treated for high blood pressure. So the preconditions were not good from the start. Many of those surveyed were also overweight. In other words, there were several risk factors that were unrelated to oestrogen supplementation.

Increasingly, medical opinion is that the results of the WHI study are not necessarily applicable to healthy women who start taking oestrogen in their forties. There is also another study worth mentioning, and that is an eighteen-year follow-up of the women in the WHI study. It showed that the risk of death from, for example, heart and vascular disease was no greater in the group taking oestrogen than in the one that took the placebo.

For me, everything became clearer when I spoke to the renowned Professor Tord Naessén at Uppsala University, who is regarded as the most knowledgeable person about oestrogen in Sweden. After our conversation, I finally understood what oestrogen is all about. He spoke positively about the role of hormone treatment in women after the menopause. He believes that, thanks to more thorough analyses and results, views on oestrogen are fortunately beginning to change. Naessén told me that several new studies show that oestrogen has a strong protective effect against heart disease, which means that it even decreases the risk of women dying during the treatment period compared to women given the placebo. According to these studies, the risk of suffering heart and vascular problems is almost halved when undergoing hormone treatment.

Therefore, with Naessén's wise thoughts and explanations behind me, I feel that it's time to stick my neck out and say that oestrogen may be good for you. According to Naessén, there are clear signs that oestrogen can decrease mortality by up to 30 to 40 per cent if you start treatment within ten years of entering the menopause. This sounds amazing, but I was of course interested in his views of starting on oestrogen as early as the perimenopause. The answer was as I thought. If you suffer from severe peri-menopausal symptoms you should consider hormone treatment, since it's the most effective and best-document-ed therapy. And his answer to the question of how long the treatment should be was that it depends who you asked. If you asked him, he would reply: for as long as you need.

This was completely revolutionary to me. More and more evidence points to hormones being able to prolong life and improve health. Why don't the media write about this research, which could influence women's lives for the better?

## HRT is no more dangerous than other lifestyle factors

Despite the documented protective effects of oestrogen, there are disadvantages, as there are with all medical treat-ments. For example, I recently read an interesting summary in the Swedish book *Menopause – An Update*, by Anna-Clara Spetz Holm, Lena Johansson and Mats Hammar. This book is intended first and foremost for primary-care physicians and doctors, but also for gynaecologists, nurs-es, midwives and student doctors. The authors wrote:

---

In summary, a combined oestrogen and progesterone treatment (HRT) has been associated with a somewhat increased risk of breast cancer. The increased risk is of the same size as for many other lifestyle factors, such as delayed first pregnancy, and remains moderate even after long-term treatment.

---

The words 'as for many other lifestyle factors' stuck with me. They made me wonder if it would be better, for example, to stop eating red meat or to quit smoking and take oestrogen instead. Everything we do in life has advantages and disadvantages. All our choices affect how we feel and I believe there are other lifestyle factors more dangerous than oestrogen. Just compare it to smoking – even if cigarettes make you feel good in the moment, they're proven to be dangerous.

One thing you have to bear in mind is that media often present us with scaremongering headlines. In August 2019, a new meta-study was released, and of course the media did almost exactly what they did 2002 after the WHI study. They terrified us with headlines like: 'Breast cancer risk of HRT is twice what was thought' or 'HRT raises breast cancer risk by third'. I bet some women just threw their patches away. Because breast cancer is something we really, really fear.

But the fact that there *is* a slight risk of breast cancer when taking HRT is not something new. It is associated with one extra case among 1,200 women treated each year. But this study should have been explained by a medical professional before it hit the headlines. It is a meta-study and should of course be interpreted as such – in other words, it is the synthesis of fifty-eight separate studies that were carried out between 1992 and 2018. What we have to understand is that in some of these studies they used a form of HRT that is no longer practised. And also that the risk of developing breast cancer by taking HRT is no greater than the risk factors associated with drinking alcohol or being overweight.

Nor does the reporting, or the study, refer to the benefits of HRT for women. The number-one killer for women is heart disease, not breast cancer. And new studies demonstrate that HRT protects the heart. With HRT the risk of experiencing heart disease decreases by at least 40 per cent. So if we stay with the evidence, this is how it is: there is a small increased risk of breast cancer by taking HRT, but a great chance of decreasing heart disease.

So overall it is your choice. I just want you to have the facts.

It is my personal belief that we are unnecessarily frightened of oestrogen. Think of it as a lifestyle factor and maybe the decision will be easier to make. Also remember that you have no idea of what the future holds. Who knows, I might get breast cancer in a couple of years or I may live to be 120. Or I might get run over by a car tomorrow. The only certainty is that we will die one day.

Generally, you could say that the negative medical attitude towards oestrogen is diminishing. More and more gynaecologists recommend taking oestrogen supplements. I believe that attitudes have changed partly because of the studies made after that of the WHI, and partly thanks to the advance of bioidentical oestrogen. It is, after all, just like the body's own and therefore works well. But although bioidentical oestrogen has become more common, it's not something new: it was available as early as the 1970s but has not had its breakthrough until now.

## Oestrogen pioneer Mirjam Furuhjelm

We owe a lot to a woman who was known as the oestrogen pioneer in Swedish gynaecology, Mirjam Furuhjelm. As early as the end of the 1960s, she started recommending oestrogen supplements in line with her conviction that, as long as a woman is alive, she should make her life as healthy and as good as possible. She herself started taking oestrogen in her fifties and lived to be ninety-four.

In the book *Blood, Sweat and Tears* by the journalist Lena Katarina Swanberg there is a wonderful passage where Mirjam Furuhjelm draws a parallel between hormonal disruption and diabetes:

---

**Well, it's common sense. A person with diabetes needs additional insulin. She whose ovaries no longer work needs additional oestrogen. And what's more, I would rather feel really well for five years than live ten years like a dog.**

---

On the question of what she thought about the recommendation that HRT should only be a short-term treatment, Mirjam countered: 'Do these people believe the functioning of the ovaries will return afterwards?'

*Blood, Sweat and Tears* was released in 2003 and was very critical of oestrogen supplementation. And of course in the years following the WHI study, the mood was very much against HRT for women. But the interesting thing is that, despite the prevailing mood, Mirjam stood her ground throughout her career, convinced that oestrogen was something good. She also spoke widely about the importance of oestrogen to our mental health. 'It's idiotic that oestrogen's advantages to mental health are not emphasised more in the debate,' she says in Swanberg's book.

And I am inclined to agree. Why doesn't anyone talk about how important oestrogen is for making us feel less down, low and depressed? Would increased uptake of oestrogen be the end for the advocates of antidepressant medicines? Is that why no one dares? But it is difficult to know which came first, the chicken or the egg. As I said before, I believe that lack of sleep is the root of all evil. Oestrogen influences the sleep hormone positively and enables us to sleep; and when we sleep better, we start to feel better again.

I will end this chapter with yet another quote from Mirjam:

If the body doesn't produce insulin, the illness is called diabetes. Without vitamin C, the body develops an illness called rickets. If a gland stops producing oestrogen, the body begins its journey into senility. It's just as appropriate that the gynaecologist gives a middle-aged woman oestrogen as it is that an optician suggests reading glasses.

---

If and when you take oestrogen is entirely your own decision. The most important thing is that you have enough knowledge to make the right decision; absorb information from different angles and don't trust blindly what one person or another says, then you will be able to choose whether or not to jump onto the hormone bandwagon. My hope is that what I have told you might help you on your way. Don't forget that it is you who gets to decide what to do for your own body.

**Fatigue:** hormonal imbalances may result in sudden and often overwhelming feelings of weakness, exhaustion and reduced energy levels that can leave you emotionally and mentally drained.

# 12

# Don't Skip the Progesterone

'I find hormones difficult to understand. When I took bioidentical progesterone cream, I started sleeping again, but my best friend did not feel well at all using it. What should I do?'

**CAMILLA, THIRTY-NINE**

Do you remember me talking about the dance between hormones? That the hormones, just like the characters in *Dirty Dancing*, must be synchronised, otherwise nothing works? The hormonal worries we experience when they are a little at loggerheads are not fun. I have also mentioned that oestrogen shouldn't be taken without progesterone. In this chapter I will talk about progesterone as a complement but also about a type of progesterone that may be taken on its own without oestrogen.

## Combining oestrogen with progesterone

A synthetic form of progesterone, called progestin, is often found in the contraceptive pill. One of the side effects of the contraceptive pill is said to be melancholy, which can be traced to this particular intake of progestin. Therefore many people choose to take the minipill instead, which contains a lower dose of progestin than the normal contraceptive pill.

During the perimenopause, symptoms such as sleeping problems and melancholy are not the result of having too much progesterone in your body, but rather *not having enough*. You could say that it is because of insufficient levels of progesterone that we feel worse – or, more accurately, because of an imbalance between oestrogen and progesterone, since it's the progesterone that starts to decrease first.

Now you may wonder why you can't just add more progesterone if progesterone levels decrease before oestrogen levels. For some reason, Swedish gynaecologists normally only prescribe progesterone as a part of a combined HRT treatment. It's still a relatively unexplored area and, since there are no major studies to suggest that this would be enough to start with, it's not recommended today.

The tips I have already given on how you can find a cure for your problems through lifestyle changes are very useful when the hormonal imbalance is at an early stage. But when hormone levels really drop to a low level, it might be time to start thinking about adding oestrogen and progesterone. As I mentioned earlier, they are both part of an HRT treatment. I have also mentioned that bioidentical oestrogen is to be preferred over the synthetic form. The same applies to progesterone.

Several studies confirm that bioidentical progesterone is preferred by the body. As early as 2005, a French study of over 80,000 women showed clearly that the risk of breast cancer increased in the group taking synthetic progesterone, but no heightened risk was found with patients given natural progesterone.

During the last few years, creams containing bioidentical

progesterone have arrived on the market. They can be ordered online and have made a large and positive breakthrough, not least thanks to Mia Lundin, a Swedish midwife who lives in the US but also works in Sweden. Mia has made women feel better with bioidentical hormones and recommends, among other things, progesterone cream. Progesterone cream isn't approved by the FDA but is considered an 'alternative' method. Many women say that using it has helped them to sleep and calmed down the wound-up feeling in their bodies.

Although gynaecologists do not always recommend it, today many women use bioidentical progesterone cream before they start taking oestrogen, in other words *not* as part of combined HRT. I have done this myself. The cream is applied where your skin is thin – I normally put it on the inside of my underarms or thighs. Dosage is difficult to state, because how much to use is very individual.

When I began using the cream, I became incredibly calm and sleepy. For a long time my body had felt hyper, the way you do when hormones start to become unbalanced. My gynaecologist told me that my experience was similar to descriptions from her other patients. Suddenly you feel calm, the worry in your body disappears, and your sleep is improved. But she also told me that progesterone cream is a hot topic in her profession, since many patients use it without understanding how it works or what its effects might be. What gynaecologists object to above all is that there have been no studies to show that progesterone cream provides adequate protection to the endometrium, which means they will not recommend it as a progesterone complement in an HRT treatment.

Having made all the lifestyle changes I have described – taking melatonin, trying progesterone cream and sometimes using Atarax – I finally came to the point where none of this was quite enough to rid me of my problems. I started approaching the menopause. At that point, my gynaecologist agreed that I should stop everything (apart from the positive lifestyle changes) and try HRT.

As a progesterone complement to my oestrogen treatment, I chose a hormone coil that works like a normal contraceptive but also releases progesterone locally which protects the endometrium. It is, however, a synthetic progesterone. I chose the coil since I am worried about feeling low (as many people are with the contraceptive pill). But if it's only released locally the risk of side effects, such as feeling down, is minimal. If there was an alternative bioidentical progesterone in the form of a coil to protect the endometrium, I would choose that instead.

## Conflicting advice

I could not stop wondering why gynaecologists had such differences of opinion. For example, my sister-in-law's gynaecologist considered progesterone cream to be an American PR stunt and insisted that it should definitely not be used. The gynaecologist of a close friend said that the notion of bioidentical progesterone being better than synthetic was nonsense – there were no proven grounds for such a claim. Ask your friends what their gynaecologists say about progesterone and you will be surprised. Everyone says different things.

It was incredibly liberating when a gynaecologist admitted on prime-time TV that not everyone in the business had the time to keep track of the latest research. In other words, maybe not all gynaecologists know that hormone symptoms can be kept in check for a couple of years with progesterone-only cream before the need to pull out the big HRT toolbox?

If you decide to take hormones, I believe that it is better to choose those which are largely reminiscent of the body's own rather than synthetic equivalents. There are several studies that show how well bioidentical progesterone interacts with bioidentical oestrogen, and that this is the best combination for women, with the least risk of side effects. Perhaps it's time the medical profession takes current research on board? It may be new and modern, and it may not be what they were taught at medical school several years ago, but everything points to it being what is best for us.

**Hair loss and brittle nails:** some women find that hormonal fluctuations cause their nails to become brittle, and others will experience hair loss.

# 13

# Look Outside Yourself

'I honestly thought it was just me. I was convinced I was going mad. Only when I confessed to my friends did I realise we were all going through the same thing – it was such a relief.'

**BRIDGET, FORTY-SEVEN**

It's clear that the current trend in health and wellness is aimed increasingly at looking inwards. How do *I* feel? What can I do to feel better? I completely agree. In order to understand yourself and enjoy well-being in your life, it's important to listen to yourself and to your body's signals. But I also think it's important to look *outwards*. I believe you should take yourself and your symptoms very seriously and try all the methods you can to feel better and find your perimenopower, but I also want you to take a look around. Is there anything outside of yourself that can make you feel better?

## The value in sharing experiences

I myself am allergic to the kind of navel-gazing that's prevalent today and I am convinced that, far from closing ourselves off, people need one another to feel better. I believe we can get more out of sharing each other's experiences and knowledge than by trying to reinvent the wheel by just looking at ourselves as individuals. The solutions aren't always within ourselves. We humans must help one another.

Is there anything you can think of, aside from the advice I have given in this book, that automatically makes you feel better? Many people would probably answer that their relationship with family and friends greatly affects their well-being. There is even research that shows that the greatest happiness is achieved by helping others. Martin Luther King Jr, said something that I often come back to: 'Life's most persistent and urgent question is, what are you doing for others?'

How can we help one another through this tough period in life? With a strong, steady base within yourself, closeness to other people, and a will to look outwards, you can get as far as you want. We humans are pack animals – we are not biologically constructed to live alone – and solutions to our problems are often considerably easier to find when we assist each other.

Of course, it's important to look inwards and discover what is most suitable for you and not trust blindly in what someone else says. Seek out the signals and instincts in your own body. But when you have done that, maybe you can help someone else, simply by sharing how you feel. Maybe you will be surprised by what you find in other people's banks of experience. I know that speaking openly and vulnerably was transformative for me during the perimenopause.

Simply start talking about your perimenopausal experiences with your nearest and dearest. Imagine the strength you might find in comparing symptoms, laughing, crying and realising that life is actually pretty good if you share and dare to accept help. There is such value in having friendships and helping your friends – something that might even make you feel better than all the natural remedies, exercise sessions and oestrogen patches in the whole world.

And don't forget that this is not just something happening to you and your friends, it is actually happening to a community of women all around the globe. I have found so much comfort on social media, where there are groups and menopause warriors sharing their experiences even if they don't know each other in real life. It reminds us that we are all the same. And online friends can validate your experiences. If we women fight together for increased awareness about the perimenopause and menopause, maybe we can sort it out for the generations to come. I don't have daughters but I am doing this for my sons. They will hopefully one day get married and understand what their wives are going through thanks to our struggle. That thought gives me much comfort.

**Loss of libido:** it is hardly surprising that women in the throes of the perimenopause experience a loss of libido. But there is no need to accept this as inevitable – it is a well-known symptom of hormonal fluctuations, and you can get your mojo back.

# 14

# Your New Beginning

'Whenever I feel bad, I use that feeling to motivate me to work harder. I only allow myself one day to feel sorry for myself. When I'm not feeling my best I ask myself, "What are you gonna do about it?" I use the negativity to fuel the transformation into a better me.'

**BEYONCÉ**

One of the most important things for me, now that you have almost finished the book, is that you realise you are not alone. As well as your friends, most women you meet at work, on the bus, in the shop or at the gym also have problems at certain times of their lives. My intention is to make you understand how your body works and that what you are experiencing isn't an illness, but a temporary state that will come to an end.

Try to give your body the best preconditions possible during this time. I urge you to avoid sleeping pills and anti-depressants for as long as you can. If you get to the point where you must take them, make it a temporary choice. I believe you can really benefit from accepting where you are right now, and what is changing in your body. Don't fight it or resist it. Try to find solutions instead. We will always experience difficult and trying times throughout our lives and there is some truth in the saying, 'It's not about what you have, but how you deal with it.'

Try to find an approach that makes you see your peri-menopause and your symptoms more positively. You have a superpower within you which, at the moment, is hidden by strange symptoms. Find yourself again, for behind all the difficulties is your perimenopower, I promise.

## Assessing the science

It is clear that there will always be new medical studies on and evidence about the perimenopause and menopause as the science develops. Do be careful about how you interpret articles in the media. Just because a new study shows that evening primrose oil is effective against menopausal problems, it doesn't necessarily mean that it will help you. Even I, who work in health and media, sometimes find it difficult to choose which studies to trust. But one of the guidelines I normally follow is that the more participants in the study the better. A survey of 200,000 women is much more likely to be trustworthy than one of only 200.

There is also a big difference in the way studies are designed. A randomised controlled trial is the method that is used within medical research and is considered to be the gold standard. People are randomly assigned to one of two or more groups. One group receives the intervention (for example a new drug) and the control group receives nothing. This is even more reliable if the study is double-blinded, which means that no one knows who takes the drug, neither the participants nor the medical team.

Use your discretion when reading articles that say that 'a study shows . . .' The results and facts of the study may have been skewed or made to fit for the sake of the article, and may also derive from a minor study with just a few participants. Or perhaps the study looked at people in a far-away country with completely different diets and lifestyles from ours. The same study may have shown a completely different result if it had been conducted under different conditions and on other participants. Unfortunately, one can be certain that for every study that proves one thing, there is another that proves the opposite. In other words, you should be careful what you choose to believe. Give everything you read some extra analysis, and try to find articles from reputable sources that show similar results.

My conclusion, having studied this subject for many years, is that the health profession too easily gives perimenopausal women a diagnosis of depression or exhaustion, prescribing antidepressants or sleeping pills and sick leave. What if these women simply have a hormonal problem, and if these hormones could be sorted out, maybe the phenomenon of exhaustion would not be so widespread? What if women in their forties are not having a burnout but are instead approaching the menopause? I don't wish to belittle diagnoses of exhaustion, but I believe some women would feel so much better if their hormones were rebalanced. I think the connection is greater than anyone realises. I also think that one of the biggest problems we face is that even though the conversation about the menopause is becoming louder, we have to remember that the rockiest part of the transition is not the menopause itself, but the perimenopause.

## Make sure you get the right help

I learned a great deal during my own perimenopause and I learned even more while carrying out the research for this book. Above all, I learned not to be so quick to believe what other people say, even if they have the authority of a doctor or a health food adviser. I believe you gain more from being open to new knowledge and making your own decisions. You are, after all, the one who will have to live with those decisions in the end.

Don't automatically believe what the newspapers tell you, and do take everything that you read on the internet with a pinch of salt. True or not, there are some strange studies out there. And don't believe the scaremongering that oestrogen is dangerous, for there are just as many studies that show it to be vital to the long-term health of older women.

If you go to your doctor and feel that you are not receiving the right kind of help, ask to be referred to a gynaecologist. In my opinion, the doctor should refer you to one from the start. I had an interesting discussion with a close friend of mine, a doctor at a local medical centre, about how he dealt with this type of problem. He could see a connection between hormonal issues and signing people off work sick. Today he refers his patients to a gynaecologist, and the incidence of sick leave has decreased markedly. However, I do think this kind of action is rare. Once you have been referred to a gynaecologist, it's important that you feel comfortable with him or her. Should you feel misunderstood, you can hopefully change to another one.

Life is a gift. Seize every minute. It's not about *being given* help for your symptoms, it's about *going out and getting* help. Now that you know more about how your body works, you have the power. Don't sit and wait; instead get help if you think that you need it. Finally, I would like to share a mantra that I like: 'Life is not a dress rehearsal – this is probably it. Make it count.'

I try to live that way as much as I can. I try to be grateful and not become overwhelmed with things. I try to realise that I have a superpower, and constantly remind myself of it. I also think about how we shouldn't worry so much, that maybe we should be more relaxed about things. As far as I know, this is the only life we have. Try to make the best of it, even if it feels that things are sometimes going against you. Give yourself the best preconditions and you will see that everything will be OK.

I hope you find your perimenopower, as I found mine.

'We have pain on a cycle for years and years and years and then, just when you feel you are making peace with it all, what happens? The menopause comes, the f***ing menopause comes, and it is the most wonderful f***ing thing in the world. And yes, your entire pelvic floor crumbles and you get f***ing hot and no one cares, but then you're free, no longer a slave, no longer a machine with parts. You're just a person.

Phoebe Waller-Bridge, *Fleabag: The Scriptures*, (Hodder & Stoughton, 2019)

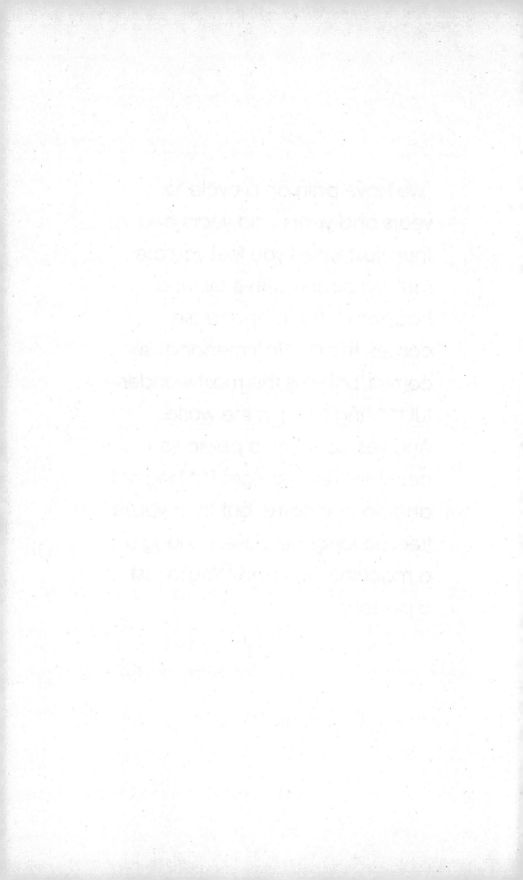

# Thank You

Thank you for reading this book, it was written for you. If you'd like to share your own experiences, there are many of us who would like to hear them. Please use the hashtag #perimenopower and tag me at @katarinawilk so that, together, we can make even more women understand that they are not alone in the chaos of the perimenopause.

Thank you, Ehrlin Publishing, for believing in my idea. Thanks to Elin Westerberg, my editor, who has been a rock throughout this whole process. You have given me invaluable advice! Another person who has been invaluable is Doctor Evelina Sande Idenfeldt. Without you there would never have been a book. I would also like to take the opportunity to thank the other doctors who have allowed me to interview them, and especially Doctor Margareta Nordenvall, whom I myself have been seeing for several years.

I would also like to express my gratitude to Orion Spring and my UK publisher, Pippa Wright, who chose to publish the book in English.

Thanks to my sisters, Monica and Anna, who have supported me the entire way. Your support, when I have been struck by self-doubt, has meant so much.

Thanks also to my fantastic friends – none mentioned, none forgotten. Thanks for putting up with me, for listening and believing in me and making me feel loved and appreciated.

I especially want to thank my sons, Ville and David, who have been forced to listen for such a long time to my ramblings on a subject which isn't at the top of the list for teenage boys. Thank you for being there. You are the light in my life. I would be nothing without you.

And last, but not least, thank you, Mum and Dad, for teaching me never to stop dreaming. That everything is possible as long as you want it deeply enough and work for it. I know you both applaud me from heaven.

*Katarina Wilk*

# References

Allmen, Tara (2016). *Menopause Confidential*. New York: HarperOne.

Burke, Tina M., et al. (2015). 'Effects of caffeine on the human circadian clock in vivo and in vitro'. *Science Translational Medicine*, 7(305).

Burkholder, Amy (2007, 20 January). 'Perimenopause: Hormone ups and downs can last years'. *CNN*. Retrieved from http://edition.cnn.com/2007/health/01/10/peri. menopause/

Collaborative Group on Hormones (2019). 'Type and timing of menopausal hormone therapy and breast cancer risk: individual participant meta-analysis of the worldwide epidemiological evidence'. *The Lancet*, epub 2019 August 29.

Davey, Gwyneth K., et al. (2003). 'EPIC-Oxford: lifestyle characteristics and nutrient intakes in a cohort of 33 883 meat-eaters and 31 546 non meat-eaters in the UK'. *Public Health Nutrition*, 6(3).

Dolgen, Ellen (2014, 22 December). 'A look at menopause through the ages'. *Huffington Post*. Retrieved from https://www.huffingtonpost.com/ellen-sarver-dolgen/history-of-menopause_b_6159614.html

Eckerman, Ingrid (2017). 'Vad ska vi äta och varför'. *AllmänMedicin, Tidskrift för svensk förening för allmänmedicin*, 3(38).

Ellenbogen, Jeffrey M. (2005). 'Cognitive benefits of sleep and their loss due to sleep deprivation'. *Neurology*, 64(7).

Fryer, Bronwyn (2006, October). 'Sleep deficit: The performance killer'. *Harvard Business Review*.

Gottfried, Sara (2015). *The Hormone Reset Diet*. New York: HarperOne.

Hammar, Mats, et al. (1990). 'Does physical exercise influence the frequency of postmenopausal hot flushes?'. *Acta Obstetricia et Gynecologica Scandinavica*, 69(5).

Harpaz, Mickey (2013, 12 October). 'The history of menopause'. *Menopause Matters*. Retrieved from http://menopausematterstoday.com/the-history-of-menopause/

Harvard Womens's Health Watch (2018, 24 August).

'Perimenopause: Rocky road to menopause'. Retrieved from https://www.health.harvard.edu/womens-health/perimenopause-rocky-road-to-menopause

Johansson, Martina (2017). *Hormonbibeln 2.0: För kvinnor genom hela livet*. Stockholm: Pagina.

Kim, Min-Ju, et al. (2014). 'Association between physical activity and menopausal symptoms in perimenopausal women'. *BMC Women's Health*.

Kirby, Julia (2013, May). 'Change the world and get to bed by 10:00'. *Harvard Business Review*.

Le, Lap Tai and Sabaté, Joan (2014). 'Beyond meatless, the health effects of vegan diets: Findings from the Adventist cohorts'. *Nutrients*.

Lee, Duck-chuul, et al. (2014). 'Leisure-time running reduces all cause and cardiovascular mortality risk'. *Journal of the American College of Cardiology*, 64(5).

Linde, Klaus, et al. (2008). 'St John's wort for major depression'. *Cochrane Database of Systematic Reviews*.

Liu, Tong-Zu, et al. (2016). 'Sleep duration and risk of all-cause mortality: A flexible, non-linear, meta-regression of 40 prospective cohort studies'. *Sleep Medicine Reviews*, 32.

Lundin, Mia (2011). 'Kaos i kvinnohjärnan'. *The Center for*

# References

*Hormonal and Nutritional Balance Inc.*

Lundin, Mia (2012, 1 November). 'Samspelet mellan kvinnohormoner och signalsubstanser'. *Kostrådgivarna*. Retrieved from http://www.kostradgivarna.se/2012/11/samspelet-mellan-kvinnohormoner-och-signalsubstanser/

Makara-Studzinska, Marta, et al. (2014). 'Epidemiology of the symptoms of menopause – an intercontinental review'. *Menopause Review/Przeglqd Menopauzalny*, 13(3).

Mandal, Ananya (2013, 2 December). 'What are hormones?' *News Medical Life Sciences*. Retrieved from https://www.news-medical.net/health/What-are-Hormones.aspx

Manson, JoAnn E., et al. (2017). 'Menopausal hormone therapy and long-term all-cause and cause-specific mortality: The Women's Health Initiative randomized trials'. *JAMA*, 318(10) .

Minkin, Mary Jane and Wright, Carol V. (2005). *A Woman's Guide to Menopause and Perimenopause*. New Haven and London: Yale University Press.

Nayak, Gavathry, et al. (2014). 'Effect of yoga therapy on physical and psychological quality of life of perimenopausal women in selected coastal areas of Karnataka, India'. *Journal of Mid-Life Health*, 5(4).

Somers, Suzanne (2013). *I'm Too Young for This!: The*

*Natural Hormone Solution to Enjoy Perimenopause*. New York: Harmony Books.

Spetz Holm, Anna-Clara, et al. (2014). *Klimakteriet – en uppdatering*. Lund: Studentlitteratur.

Stenholtz, David (2017). 'Vegansk kost – många fördelar finns men kunskap krävs'. AllmänMedicin, *Tidskrift för svensk förening för allmänmedicin*, 3(38).

Sternfeld, Barbara and Dugan, Sheila (2001). 'Physical activity and health during the menopausal transition'. *Obstetrics and Gynecology Clinics*, 38(3).

Swanberg, Lena Katarina (2003). *Blod, svett och tårar: En ilsken bok om östrogen*. Stockholm: Bokförlaget DN.

# Interviews

Torbjörn Åkerstedt, Professor of Psychology at Karolinska Institutet. Email interview, January 2018.

Mats Hammar, Professor Emeritus of Obstetrics and Gynaecology at Linköping University. Email interview, November 2017.

Evelina Sande Idenfeldt, Chief Physician of Obstetrics and Gynaecology. Continuous phone interviews, September 2017 to February 2018.

Tord Naéssen, Professor of Obstetrics and Gynaecology at Uppsala University. Phone interview, January 2018.

# Useful websites:

www.menopause.org
www.whi.org
www.imsociety.org

# About the Author

Katarina Wilk is a Swedish writer and journalist, specialising in health and lifestyle subjects. As a child she dreamed of becoming a doctor, and she turned this passion for medicine into a career writing about wellness and the ways in which we can all improve our lives. Her personal experience of the perimenopause led her to investigate how women can best navigate their way through this hormonal transition.

# Help us make the next generation of readers

We – both author and publisher – hope you enjoyed this book. We believe that you can become a reader at any time in your life, but we'd love your help to give the next generation a head start.

Did you know that 9 per cent of children don't have a book of their own in their home, rising to 13 per cent in disadvantaged families*? We'd like to try to change that by asking you to consider the role you could play in helping to build readers of the future.

We'd love you to think of sharing, borrowing, reading, buying or talking about a book with a child in your life and spreading the love of reading. We want to make sure the next generation continue to have access to books, wherever they come from.

And if you would like to consider donating to charities that help fund literacy projects, find out more at **www.literacytrust.org.uk** and **www.booktrust.org.uk**.

THANK YOU

*As reported by the National Literacy Trust